Blood Mysteries

by

Gillian Macdonald

GREEN
MAGIC

Blood Mysteries © 2013 by Gillian Macdonald.
All rights reserved.
No part of this book may be used or reproduced in any form without written permission of the author, except in the case of quotations in articles and reviews.

Green Magic
5 Stathe Cottages
Stathe
Somerset
TA7 0JL
England
info@greenmagicpublishing.com
www.greenmagicpublishing.com

Typeset by Green Man Books, Dorchester
www.greenmanbooks.co.uk

ISBN 978-0-9566197-2-3

GREEN MAGIC

Religion was born of blood and has bathed in blood ever since, this is the sacrament.

Dedicated to the memory of Cain — I only had you for one year but you were the most awesome cat I've ever been privileged to love.

Acknowledgements

Thanks firstly to Pete Gotto at Green Magic Publishing for being so patient waiting for this book to finally arrive. Thanks to Cain Helsson and Pier Ruaro for their advice, knowledge and friendship. Thanks also to John Crow for little tasty morsels on various subjects. And all my family and friends… you know who you are!

Disclaimer

No responsibility will be taken by the writers or publishers of this book should you decide to try any of the rituals described. They are intended for information only and are merely of esoteric interest.

CONTENTS

Introduction	vii
Chapter One: Menstruation and Birth	1
Chapter Two: Hunting	35
Chapter Three: Tattooing, Piercing and Scarification	57
Chapter Four: Vampires	73
Chapter Five: Human Sacrifices	91
Chapter Six: Religious Blood Rituals	121
Chapter Seven: Cannibals	153
Chapter Eight: Medical	163
Suggested further reading	176

INTRODUCTION

Mention blood and many people squirm with discomfort and yet we all have around eight pints of it fuelling our systems for most of our adult lives. It is our literal essence and the blue print for our ancestry. Some people are squeamish about it, some indifferent to it and a lesser minority are actually drawn to it for a variety of reasons.

Blood mysteries open the door to taboos of all sorts, some of which might be disturbing. We will travel from the lunar links with women's mysteries to tribal tattooing and hunting rituals, to the morbid practices of live sacrifices. The nocturnal world of Vampires and the true origins of this legend will be explored, as will the less supernatural medical blood rites. We will look into esoteric and sexual blood rites/rituals opening up doors for future development and thought-provoking, yet challenging conversations.

Blood fascinates many of us, often for varying reasons. With the quite justified fear and controversy surrounding some of the practises written about in this book it is understandable that, in some cases, misnomers occur.

Some of these rites might shock, some may well revolt and some could just could excite you. I will say that all blood rites involve both legal implications and health risks so I have highlighted these. It is therefore up to you, as discriminating adults, to make your own decisions regarding them.

As the majority of people who read this book are likely to be pagan or have an interest in the occult or esoteric world, I have tried to find direct information connected to blood and our spiritual and religious evolution.

The book begins with an exploration into menstruation and birth, two virtually inescapable female attributes. Myths and superstitions abound in nearly every culture regarding this feminine cycle, and it seems many of our ancestors were less uncomfortable about it than we are today. Indeed, it seems to be one aspect of being female that is more supressed in this so called 'modern day society in the West' than many others. Whilst looking at the ways in which other cultures have dealt with and viewed it, I was dismayed to find our current thinking seems to be devolving where menses is concerned. Birth is one of the most emotive rites of passage we go through. Whether it is our own birth or watching our children born or the mother giving birth, nothing apart from death comes close to the passions it fuels.

The act of giving birth also goes through fads and fashions, with constant changes being made to the way we deal with it. Since the establishment of maternity suites in NHS hospitals, many mothers have automatically been sent to them when in labour, thinking that having the support network of that 'safe' environment is for the best. Such conditions are only recentlybeing realised to be retarded in their thinking, with the mother now being offered whatever option she might find most relaxing to enable her birthing experience to be easier. It seems that we who have been born into this technological age are slowly seeing how the recent traditions actually work against the natural process. Over the last thirty years, a slow return to natural birthing has occurred. The medical and technical services are still there as back-up, but allowing mothers the chance to opt out of the clinical route if there are no complications is a step forward.

From this I go on to examine hunting. Hunting has been a part of human life for much longer than we originally thought. New evidence from anthropologists and archaeologists is proving that even homo-erectus, a precursor to the homo-sapiens who lived among us for some time before finally dying out, hunted with rudimentary tools and even cooked meat on fires. This takes such activities back to well over 1.5 million years ago, a number that few of us can really comprehend. So hunting is a very ancient skill indeed, but discovering ancient blood rites and rituals surrounding it is difficult as we only have a few thousand years of written recorded human history. However, traditions often out live people and are carried on, so many that are still carried out today might well have their roots in much older practises. It amazes me that hunting was a daily occurrence, and still is for a minority, and yet today most of us have never experienced it or ever will. But I believe the ancestral knowledge is instinctual in many of us and should necessity arise, we could all do it if we had to.

From hunting, we continue into the world of tattooing and permanent scarification. It is entirely possible and probable that these arts and rituals also have their roots in very ancient practises that we are unlikely to ever really know about. Deliberately cutting the skin to leave a mark or scar seems primal and, as such, can get us in touch with a spiritual link that might go back many hundreds of thousands of years. Evidence from mummies and well-preserved ancient bodies shows us that many cultures practised one or more types of tattooing and scarification. I will look at modern day tattooing as well as tribal customs and both religious and superstitious beliefs surrounding it.

Next, we visit the nocturnal world of the Vampyre or Vampire (depending on your view). This creepy character has seeped into our minds mainly through modern-day popularity and the film industry but has its roots in folklore from many parts of the world. I explore the origins of Dracula and the Vampire myths. From the alleged bloody crimes of Countess de Bathory to a modern day cult of Vampires no bloody subject holds quite so much fascination for us. The blood drinking immortal has very little to do with it though and for those hoping for romanticism and castles hanging from precarious cliffs, I've done my best — but the truth is weirder.

And then we travel onto Human Sacrifices, and how the concept of them evolved over time in most cultures and religions. We visit South America and the ancient mysterious worlds of the Aztecs and Mayans among others. Here we see how this bloody aspect of their everyday life was constantly hanging over them as remnants of past victims are permanently displayed and incorporated into their architecture and art. Travelling back to the African continent, we are suddenly in the world of human muti-killings and we see how these might have spread to the UK.

Cannibalism has occurred for varying reasons in many cultures throughout time. And it might come as a surprise to some to hear that it is still happening today. Some of these practices are described and the cannibal's motives examined. We go from religious motivation to cold blooded murder and a taste for human flesh to the ultimate desperation of starvation.

Then we look at more specific religious blood rituals and rites from the Abrahamic paths, to ancient pagan ones and modern day vodhun/voodoo. This particular journey was taken with a desire for a greater understanding of how differing paths and traditions have managed to keep some of these rituals alive today. We touch upon Hindu ones to Kali, Native American ones now outlawed, and modern day rituals you can still take part in should you wish to.

And lastly, we examine the history of blood in the Western medical world. Here we discover the Egyptians at the literal cutting edge of science way back several thousand years ago and move forward to modern day practises. We look at the history of blood transfusion and heart surgery.

This is a concise introduction to some of the subject matters touched upon. I have tried to keep the topics on aspects I considered might be of most interest to people from all walks of life, but make no apology for the fact that the book does have a pagan and esoteric onus. This is especially evident in the rituals at the end of some of the chapters.

In these dangerous days of HIV, Hepatitis C and AIDS plus other less dangerous contaminations we have to be aware that blood has become way more frightening a substance to have contact with. The risk of catching something deadly through direct blood to blood contamination is much higher than it was thirty or so years ago. But even though this is a known fact, and sexual education highlights it — as do doctors and hospitals, people still take risks. My opinion is that it is up to each of us to take responsibility for our own health and the potential risk we can pose to others.

The Callings

At the end of some chapters, I have included a calling to a specific deity connected with the energy of the topic covered. These callings are intended as informative rather than for practical use. This book isn't describing any particular tradition or one purely of witchcraft and therefore the callings can, in theory, be adapted to suit several paths. These are not direct examples of ancient rites and are more in keeping with modern neo-pagan formats. I have only included callings to deities I am familiar with. I don't think it right to use other peoples rituals without permission and decided to stick with my own.

For this reason I have avoided giving a step by step detailed format as this book will be read by people from varying paths and traditions, each with their own methods and constructs for creating ritual.

Some magical traditional paths have an extremely precise formula and if yours is one such type, it is definitely best to stick to the guidance of your magister or mentor and the spells and rites as prescribed for you.

CHAPTER ONE
Menstruation and Birth

This book had to start somewhere and I make no apology for it beginning here. It seemed to me when first contemplating writing a book on blood mysteries that menstruation and birth is where it all begins, for all of us. Our first contact with blood is not remembered. It is the direct nourishment we all receive from the placenta in the womb and is, therefore, our most commonly shared blood rite. But before this can happen we need to journey back a bit further and look at menstruation.

There are very few women in the world who find their first bloodletting an entirely positive and comfortable experience. And I'm not just talking about the physical experience. Most girls feel different, strange and ungrounded leading up to it and this is the mildest of emotions attached to menses; the full spectrum can range from excited to deep depression, to anger and pretty much everything else in between. All their senses are heightened, their intuition goes through the roof and their ability to remain calm alongside their fellow men diminishes as women prepare to hide, to cave, to retreat. When a girl sees that blood flow from between her legs for the first time it is unsettling, primal, weird, and fearful, yet fascinating. It marks a massive shift in a girls life and is the conformation that she is now a fertile woman, in theory, and able to have children. Her body has been giving her all sorts of signals as her hormones increase. Sexual urges are being born and explored, often in secret to begin with, before she takes it that step further. And for some, the pain that goes hand in hand with this next stage of life is also a shock or unpleasant surprise. Most women will go from their own birth to menstruating, to pregnancy and giving birth at least once in their life. Not all do, admittedly, but the majority do. And men will, for the most part, see this as a bit of a mystery.

The origin of menses or menstruation comes from a word that springs from the Greek *menus* meaning monthly power. Monthly power it is but it has since been relegated as a curse upon women, and as each generation of mothers bemoans their menstrual cramps and complains about the monthly bleed so the negative association is imprinted upon the emotional psyche. Now very few women in the Western world view it in an entirely positive light. They plug it up, cover it up and camouflage any potential aroma with artificial scents lest they be discovered to be 'on'.

And yet it wasn't that long ago in our recorded history that some cultures embraced it as a sign of health and fertility and a blessing. They cared less about that particular body odour. Up until the arrival of disposable sanitary items women made their own pads or simply bled and let the flow, well, flow. It has only really been over the last one hundred years that we have sought to sanitise to such a degree. We seem to have arrived at a point where all natural odours are now covered up. Even modern sanitary towels are impregnated with deodoriser lest anyone get even a subconscious whiff of blood.

Modern Homo sapiens in their current form have been living on this planet for over 200,000 years. We have no idea what views, traditions and cultural variances there were relating to menses prior to the creation of recorded history, so we only have the last few thousand years to go on. It does seem, however, that during this time our attitude and reaction towards menstruation has always had some form of stigma attached to it. We still, to this day, shroud it in a mysterious veil choosing to avoid talking about it by and large. And yet without that precious life creating blood none of us would be here. Our ancient female ancestors bled in just the same way as we do. It was and still is a sign of potential fertility. This mysterious ability all healthy fertile women have to bleed for several days without dying was one of their most magical and potent mysteries. And one of the earliest coincidences ever noticed was the parallel between the moons monthly cycle and women's ones. It's not clear if our Paeolithic and Neolithic hunter gatherer ancestors had made this link. Nor is it always the case with the subsequent pagan religions. If they saw the Goddess as lunar it might be fair to say the direct influence was believed in. For those who saw the moon as a God perhaps they believed that the god inflicted the cycle upon women. But when you start counting them it seems there were more Goddesses linked with the moon than Gods, which leads us to think that the lunar cycle and that of the woman's menstrual one not only had a mystical relationship to many in the ancient civilised world, but perhaps had one way before then also.

The average gap between periods is between 21-28 days, and the moon's cycle is roughly 28. Though it is rare for any woman to actually synchronise exactly with the moon's phases, the symbolic and spiritual waxing and waning of the fertile cycle was comparative. Modern day pagans and Wiccans like to see this as representative of the maid phase. The period between new and full is coupled with the ripening and readiness of the woman to conceive and when she has opened up to be fertile. The full moon is also representative in many early cultures with the full belly of the pregnant woman. The waning phase was often linked with crone goddesses or old age and, though it didn't have a direct link with the menstrual cycle, it falls during the period where uncertainty lies — is the woman pregnant or not? The dark of the moon is linked with menstruation in many ancient societies and in many subsequent shamanic and pagan beliefs.

Early examples of Goddesses with lunar links can be found all over the world in names such as Hekate from Greece, Cheng-O from China, Mawa from Dahomey Africa, Luna from Ancient Rome, Cerridwen from Celtic Wales, Isis from Egypt, Lilith or Ishtar from Babylonia, Ix-Chel from Mayan South America… the list goes on and on… there are hundreds of ancient moon Goddesses. And this in itself speaks volumes.

Although it is most likely that mankind's earliest spiritual beliefs were born of death and the desire we have to keep a living link with our ancestors it is also possible that birth and women's mysteries came a close second. The myth that we were once all Goddess worshipping is just that, a myth. In most ancient pagan cultures both Gods and Goddesses were feared, revered and respected but there doesn't really seem to be worship. Their festivals were celebrated often by whole communities and frequently sacrificial offerings made but again, no direct evidence of worship as such. This might not go down well with those who believe we once had a global gynocracy but it is true nonetheless.

Most archaeologists and anthropologists now agree that the spiritual beliefs of most cultures throughout the Mesolithic, Neolithic and more recently the start of the Holocene world seem rooted in shamanic type practises. These paths still exist in varying forms in indigenous peoples, with each tradition having its own unique peculiarities. The majority of early societies tend to believe in some sort of creation myth. They honour their ancestors and use mediumistic techniques to commune with them. These ancestors are considered closer to petition than Gods, who are seen as distant. The emphasis of most of these early paths seems rooted in the ability of the shaman / priest to travel on astral planes and deal with both benevolent and evil spirits. Blood was and still is sometimes used as an offering to these spirits, especially if wishing to keep the connection strong between family members. And it doesn't take a massive leap in our imaginations to see that blood played an important role in the forming of our earliest spiritual beliefs. Before we sought to settle and farm, our relationship with nature was closer to the everyday bloody business of the hunt. Our blood tied us to the animal kingdom and made sure we knew our place in it.

Although each tribal culture would have its own take on menses, there are many aspects that seem to be accepted by most. This blood was seen as different from the sort that flows through our veins, which was an accurate observation. The fact that women can bleed without seeming to suffer injury or die was also seen as mystical and magical. Some cultures developed a negative superstitious view of menses, believing contact with it would take men's power from them, while some viewed it as a positive sign of fertility to be exalted. In these cases, women could also bleed without stigma or disgust or protection and it was to be celebrated and honoured and respected, even if they were segregated or limited in what they could do. Hippocrates believed that that blood fermented inside a woman's body and it was due to this, and the fact they didn't sweat out as many of the impurities, that caused menstruation. Aristotle got close to reality, claiming that it was excess blood left over from creating babies. But myths and fears surrounding it perpetuated in all cultures with some seeing the blood itself as inherently toxic and harmful.

One peculiar effect that is mainly noticed in communities of both sexes is that of 'synchronous menstruation', or the apparent ability that women who spend a lot of time together have to gradually adjust their cycles to merge. In 1971 Martha McClintock published an article on menstrual synchrony in Nature magazine.

Her findings resulted in the pheromone theory, or 'McClintock effect'. The test was also carried out in a lesbian community where no discernible changes in women's cycles occurred, as opposed to those of a heterosexual nature whose cycles merged. This leads many to think that it has something to do with the subconscious competitive desire by all women to attract the alpha male genes. If they were all on the same cycle they would have to compete to have sex with the alpha, with the most dominant alpha female presumably winning.

The taboos tend to be more supernatural in origin whereas the rules are definitive and have in many cases been derived from the taboos. The practise of keeping women in menses separated from the rest of the tribe evolved and is still found to this day from Hawaii to parts of Africa. It is all too easy for those of us not familiar with this to view it in a negative light, thinking it was a punishment for women, but this is not so. As it seems a cross-cultural phenomena, there must in my eyes be a primitive reason for it. It is believed to stem from two occasionally concurrent beliefs. One is that the woman's menstrual blood is a dangerous substance in itself and to be avoided at all costs and the other is the belief that women were more magical, sacred and inspired at this time. Their sensitivity was seen as both a blessing and a curse. In many cultures that use menses huts or exclusion, the belief is that the woman's power is at its height and therefore the woman can be more of a danger to her fellow men in both a physical sense and a magical one.

In some tribes and cultures menstrual blood was collected, with the woman's permission, and used for rituals. And one that makes sympathetic sense is that of spreading the blood over fields for fertility. By keeping women in menses separate they could avoid the problem of losing it by walking about and it meant that the tribe had the magical potency of that woman's blood. The more fertile she was, the more precious her blood — the tradition may have been interpreted as some sort of sign that they were 'unclean', the women concerned are usually very happy for a monthly holiday and chance to retreat from duty. There are many religious rules that have evolved from this that control what the women can and can't eat or touch, who she can be in the company of and where she is allowed to go. There is also a lot of superstition that if a woman goes about her normal business whilst bleeding she might bring bad luck to the family or village. Most traditions encourage a ritual wash once the bleeding has ceased which makes sense really.

In this so called liberated technical age these practices sound sexist but only because we place our own modern cultural projection onto it. It is a remnant of a much older ritual or tradition and considering women do change on all levels around the time of their period, it is a shame we have suppressed this so much. I've long felt that PMT/S is probably more to do with diet and environmental factors common to the developed world. Perhaps this is also because modern women have more periods than our ancestors did. There certainly is evidence for the onset of menses to be later and lives shorter and with infant mortality higher for ancient ancestors, they spent more time pregnant than we choose to. We also have choice, by and large. Until effective contraception arrived, women in most cultures were spending more time pregnant. If they had as many pregnancy free years as us then would they also have experienced pre-menstrual problems? It is impossible to say and difficult to prove either way.

There are many contributory factors in establishing the onset and lifetime of a woman's fertile time, but for most she can generally expect to start her periods at any time from 12-18 years old and end them in mid age usually between 45-55 years of age. Trends that affect a woman's cycle are many and subtle at times. Diet, genetics, age, general health, stress, exposure to artificial oestrogens, pollution contaminates, and the contraceptive pill are all responded to and can vastly alter both fertility and menstruation cycle. If the cultural emphasis is on having big families then women will experience less periods and bleed far less over their lifetimes. There are no hard and fast rules concerning menstruation; it is a delicate balance that can easily be upset by many factors.

If you have ever wondered how women managed before modern sanitary pads and plugs arrived then, after taking a virtual tour of the Museum of Menstruation in NYC, I've concluded it was with the minimum of fuss. From evidence they have gathered and some fabulous true life stories, it transpires that women took control of their own arrangements. Most chose to make washable re-usable pads out of a variety of materials if required. It is only recently that our countryside and oceans became littered with millions upon millions of towels and tampons. Although there are many on the market that are less destructive to the environment they are not promoted enough and only those in the know tend to use them Many governments levy taxes on sanitary wear as it is still considered a luxury item and in some respects it is. I can't imagine the majority of modern women making their own DIY pads or using them. It is ironic to think that the ancient practise of taking the precious magical elixir to the fields for increased fertility has since been substituted by leaving the blood all over our polluted rubbish heaps. This speaks volumes about our changing relationship with it.

Many cultures until relatively recently expected women to bleed and, if the clothing allowed it, they simply let it flow. This might sound implausible but it isn't. A woman doesn't constantly flow, her womb contracts and pushes its contents out much in the same way as labour but to a far lesser degree. This means that it is normally an intermittent flow so as long as the woman can go to the toilet as and when she feels a cramp she is unlikely to loose too much of it to gravity. If she was in a culture that allowed for segregation then the woman could simply sit back and take it easy and not really worry too much about leaving potential trails of blood behind her. This may seem abhorrent by our standards but in essence it makes more sense. It is meant to flow. It is a cleansing and clearing bodily function.

Back deep in our pre-history, when our ancestors had to be on the watch for predators, a woman leaving a trail of blood would attract unwanted attention. This instantly makes her a danger to the rest of the family or tribe. To me this seems to be the origin of the negativity surrounding menses and might also be where the idea to isolate menstruating women originally came from.

We certainly fell foul of Christian fears surrounding menses in this country. From the Middle Ages it was considered wrongful to be intimate or get close to a menstruating woman and this 'unclean' attitude continued until just before the industrial revolution. As for the actual bleeding process itself, people were less bothered by it. In fact, by allowing nature to take her course, it was healthier and curiously sexual in spite of religious opposition. Men would be attracted by the aroma of the menses as the pheromones trigger sex hormones in men. To the inner beast it signals fertility and the reptilian brain responds to it. But they couldn't say anything about it and often wouldn't know if the woman they had just noticed and instantly fancied was having her period or not.

Letting it flow also cuts down the risk of associated infections — prior to the invention of internal tampons, there certainly hadn't been any associated toxic shock syndrome due to leaving them inside for too long. Among uncircumcised women there was less risk of yeast and bladder infections. But can you imagine a modern city business woman walking down the street risking bleeding onto the pavement as she strolled along? She probably wouldn't get too far before some well-meaning social worker had her sectioned. By today's modern sanitised standards this would be seen as a lack of self respect and mental illness. So we cover it up, hide it, ignore it, rise above it and generally do everything we can to pretend from one month to the next that it just doesn't exist.

There are so many modern day myths associated with menstruating and I want to use this opportunity to be one of many to dispel them. One is that you can't get pregnant when on your period. This isn't exactly true; though the risk is less, it is not completely safe. And strange though it may seem, some women have managed to conceive during menses. Another is that menstrual blood is dirty. It isn't, in fact blood in itself cannot be viewed as dirty, but it can carry disease and infection. A very common one is that you shouldn't go swimming on your period. This is rubbish — of course you can, there is no danger involved at all. The only potential problem is embarrassment due to leakage.

Another myth that many still believe to this day, and is enforced in many cultures, is that you should avoid sex during your period. This might have stemmed from cultures that encouraged the menses hut and separation during the period. But it is generally accepted that not only is it perfectly safe, but sex during menses is actually good for you as it helps with pain and flow and encourages the feel-good endorphins.

One myth that is most definitely a more modern concept is that the smell is disgusting and must be deodorised. This is actually quite a dangerous myth. It encourages us to use strong scents and chemicals in an area with very delicate pH levels. Using deodorants around the vagina is asking for trouble and will upset the natural acid alkaline balance. The balance is already slightly less acidic during the period, so things like bacterial vaginosis (fishy smell) can breed more easily with the help of this modern fashion. Fresh water is all that is needed to wash with, or a very mild, scent free soap. The smell is meant to be one of nature's aphrodisiacs and it is modern society which has deemed it unpleasant. A very familiar modern-day concept is that you shouldn't have oral sex when on your period. This is very much up to you and your partner; there is no health risk involved and it is, if you will excuse the pun, a matter of taste. It tastes of copper.

One myth that catches out quite a few women is that you don't have periods when you are pregnant. This isn't always the case. As a rule of thumb you don't, but some women can continue to have very light periods in their early months so if you haven't used any form of contraception and think you might be pregnant go and see your doctor and have a test just to make sure. The final myth is that all women get PMT. This is not true at all — many women don't, and those from cultures that have a traditional diet high in fish and fresh veg. and fruit fare best.

Traditional & Religious Myths

In orthodox Judaism, women are excluded. This practice even has the name *niddah*. During the week of her period and sometimes for a few days after it, she is banned from having sex or being close to her husband and during her period she must avoid touching anything that other people touch. Once she has a ritual bath and immerses herself completely she is considered clean once more.

Women who come under the Christian Eastern Orthodox Church from Greece, Russia and the Ukraine are not able to receive communion whilst on their periods. As the Eucharist is thought to be the vehicle for rising above mankind's fallen ways and lifting him or her to a higher plane and closer to God, the period is a sign of the fall from grace. And yet one is a mystical blood ritual and the other a natural bleed. Here the mystical wins over the natural, as is so often the case in religious superstitions.

Islamic women are forbidden to have sex but can get close to their husbands. They are let off from praying and attending the mosque and they don't have to obey fasting laws if they clash with their period. It is understood that women should not have unnecessary stress put on them at this time and their period is treated with respect.

The ancient Mayans also saw menstruation as a curse on women and a punishment sent to a woman if she had broken any marriage laws. They believed that the blood would become either insects or snakes which would be used in black magic sorcery. They also believed that the moon Goddess is reborn from menstrual blood. Considering women didn't used to have anywhere near as many periods as modern women do today, any woman having a period was in essence being punished for not getting pregnant.

Hindu women in southern parts of India are expected to avoid temples and domestic chores for at least the first three days of their period. They are segregated and have to use separate utensils and cups etc. for food from the rest of the family. Intimacy and sex is forbidden during this time. They are considered untouchable.

In Bali, women are isolated from others and not allowed to work or have sex during their cycle. They are expected to wear the same clothing throughout their period and never wear these same ones in a temple. She is also banned from entering a temple during her period.

In Indonesia the women are considered deceitful during their period. This has risen partly because of the desire by women to avoid telling men when they are bleeding. Any sex during this time that results in an STD is blamed on the woman for giving it to the man, while men are encouraged to pass it onto a woman who will purge it out with her period. These myths are still believed by many people, especially in Sumba.

Star Fire

It is almost impossible to write about menstrual mysteries without including Sir Laurence Gardner's theories on Star Fire.

Menstruation and Birth

Star Fire is simply another way of describing menstrual blood. His theory is that the ancient high council of Sumerian Gods, the Anunnaki, lived for thousands of years. His attempt to explain the subsequent longevity of many pre-flood deities presumes they were actually living flesh and blood human beings. He suggests that they were weaned from their mother's milk onto Star Fire, or menstrual blood, and consuming this blood on a regular basis enabled them to be almost immortal. He also claims it gave them supernatural powers including telepathy and levitation. He states that after Enlil or Yahweh sent the deluge, most of the Star Fire knowledge was lost. He also links them with the story of the angelic Nephilim. In the Old Testament we find the part in which the 'sons of God' (indicating that they were perhaps angels or demi-gods in themselves), copulated with the 'daughters of men' (indicating that they were mere mortals). This leads us to think that there were more intelligent beings than just humans alive and with us in those days.

Genesis 6:1-4 reads:

"And it came to pass, when men began to multiply on the face of the earth, and daughters were born unto them, *That the sons of God saw the daughters of men that they were fair; and they took them wives of all which they chose... There were nephilim in the earth in those days; and also after that, when the sons of God came in unto the daughters of men, and they bare children to them, the same became mighty men which were of old, men of renown.*"

The reference to Nephilim is also a quandary as it may pertain to literal 'giants', as the translated Sumerian records suggest or the gigantic aspect may well mean that they were more than just human. These possible 'superhumans' might have been viewed this way because of something different or special or magical that set them 'above' or 'apart' from the masses. They were fed bodily fluids orally after weaning from the breast but it is not clear as to what exactly thes fluids were. The hybrid offspring that resulted from the union might well have gone onto becoming many of the ancient Mesopotamian deities.

In genesis 9-4 we have a clue as to the spiritual belief's concerning the ingestion of blood. It provides instructions to partake of all green and herb and beast.

But the flesh with the life thereof, which is the blood thereof, shall ye not eat.

Here is where we find the Jewish need for kosher meat. This is meat that has had the blood drained from it. Why is blood suddenly seen as a negative thing? The Sumerian records pre-date the writing of Genesis and yet in part are a direct parallel. The Anunnaki had blood sacrifices and blood related rituals, they were the pre-cursors to Abraham's Hebrew nation and didn't have a problem with ingesting blood. Various reasons have been given over the years — some stem from health reasons while others stem from changing religious beliefs, and both are probably true. The Sumerian and Akkadian peoples are also believed to have deliberately, ritually or otherwise, ingested menstrual blood or Star Fire. This has been linked by people such as Gardner and Zecharia Sitchin to an explanation for the longevity of many of the Biblical ages given in Genesis. But this might not be true at all as the ages could well be measured in moons/months rather than years.

Menstrual blood is different to the type that flows through our veins. As well as having a higher content of minerals etc, it also contains endocrinal secretions of the pineal and pituitary glands. The *Oxford English Dictionary* describes the alchemical ability of the blood to nourish and grow a baby as "*an alchemical parallel with the transmutation into gold.*"

Gardner also observes that though the Abrahamic lineage dropped ingesting all blood, they still partook of ritual sacrifice and animal offerings which were still being made in temples during Jesus's time.

If we equate the chalice as the representation of the most holy of all grails, the womb, then it makes perfect sense. And from this he deduces that knowledge of Star Fire as a sacred life-enhancing substance continued into the classical age. As King Sargon of the Akkadian peoples travelled west he introduced art, literature and other new concepts to what would become Greece and Italy. Egypt was already onto the use of Star Fire and believed in its inherent mystical power; their culture was only ever a stone's throw from the Mesopotamian and the two cultures often traded.

The sacred prostitute, or 'scarlet woman' may well in fact have been a specially chosen (for her blood lineage) young girl whose periods had just begun. Sex wasn't on the agenda here at all, contrary to popular misconceptions. She might have been trained in the raising of Shekhina (divine feminine spiritual energy) and made the offering of her menstrual blood each month for rich and powerful men and women to ingest to empower them and increase their health and even intuitive faculties. These priestesses would have been kept as healthy as possible and probably had access to the best food and accommodation, paid for by their clients. And this might also be the origin of the vestal virgins and subsequent 'brides of Christ' or nuns of today.

The practise died out with the fall of the Sumerian civilisation. And so the star fire legacy seemed to die out with it. But Gardner also sets out to prove that those still wishing to partake of this elixir made a parallel between menstrual blood and gold. He says that thanks to Tubal-Cain and the discovery of metallurgy, it became a secret practise among a certain bloodline or family to both heat and spin gold to create a white powder that has the same alchemical properties as Star Fire once did. Sales of what is now called 'white powder gold' have become very popular since his exposé as people are keen to try anything that might heal them, keep them healthy and increase their age. It seems that as blood sacrifices diminished and sacred whores fell out of fashion and the former pagan world gave way to Judaism, Christianity and Islam, so blood-related sacred activities in the Middle East also declined.

Sacred prostitution has never been definitively proved in any ancient near-eastern cultures even though many urban myths are born of it. Many scholars who have studied and translated ancient cuneiform texts say that a form of 'Sacred Marriage' often occurred between Sumerian kings and the High Priestess Inanna, Sumerian goddess of sexual love, fertility, and war. Interestingly enough there is no absolute evidence that sexual intercourse was included. It is this ritual that might well have been the Star Fire ceremony as researched by Gardner.

The Jewish Bible uses two different words for 'prostitute', *zonah* and *kedeshah*. The word *zonah* applies to an ordinary prostitute or lady of the street. But the word *kedeshah* literally means 'consecrated (feminine form)', from the Semitic origin, *q-d-sh*, that means 'holy' or 'set apart'. We have already seen the term 'set apart' in relation to women menstruating and it most definitely means to segregate. This would also make sense if temple prostitution was less to do with sex and more to do with blood donation. The Jewish Bible makes it clear that any form of ritual, religious prostitution had no place in Judaism. And in Deuteronomy 23:18-19 we find...

None of the daughters of Israel shall be a kedeshah, nor shall any of the sons of Israel be a kadesh. You shall not bring the hire of a prostitute (zonah) or the wages of a dog (keleb) into the house of the Lord your God to pay a vow, for both of these are an abomination to the Lord your God.

If such titles were wound up in the sacred blood ritual then it also makes sense that it would be prohibited by the Hebrew beliefs and religious instructions as laid down in the Old Testament. Though it is easy to imagine the females role in such acts and not quite so simple to apply this potential connection to the male 'kadesh'. It is possible that men did play some sort of ceremonial role in the temple during this ritual that might not have been directly involved in the 'set apart' ritual going on with the women involved. This is speculation does seem to fit rather well.

Female Genital Mutilation (FGM)

One blood rite that horrifies many of us whose culture and society haven't ever practised it is Female Genital Mutilation, or FGM. These forms of circumcision are gradually being made illegal in many cultures and countries but it is estimated that up to 140 million women alive today have had some type of FGM carried out on them. There doesn't seem to be any one particular religion that advocates it as such even though many associate it with Islamic tradition, this is not so.

The Jewish people may still practise male circumcision but have banned the female type as unnecessary and against human rights. The WHO, or World Health Organisation, is making slow progress with some countries placing pressure on them to ban it as a major health risk. At least 10% of girls who have one of these procedures done will die from secondary complications and infections due to the surgery.

Trying to find the origins of the practice is difficult. There is evidence on Egyptian mummies for it leading many to think it originated here but not all female mummies have it. There is also evidence that ancient Romans practised it, but again, not on all women. But one possible cause for it seems to be rooted in slavery. Many of the countries with cultures that still practise it regardless of religion are African, Indonesian and Middle Eastern. All have history of their people at some time or another being taken and used as slaves. It proved a very useful way of preventing slave girls from getting pregnant. This is especially so with type four mutilations.

There are four basic types of FGM. The first, and most

common, is where the tip of the clitoris is removed. This is meant to lessen the female libido.

The second one is more severe and the entire bud and hood is removed.

The third includes the removal of the inner labia as well as the clitoris. This is also to reduce female libido.

In the fourth and most severe, the entire outer and inner labia plus the whole clitoris is removed, and then the area is sewn up only allowing for a tiny hole for urine and another for menstrual blood to escape. This sort is the one most associated with diseases and many varieties of complication. This one is to remove libido, to keep the intact appearance of virginal status, and to stop any woman from being unfaithful to her husband. The vagina area has to be cut open for her husband to have sex and sewn back up again afterwards. It is also re-opened for each birth. This severe trauma can lead to such heavy thickening of the area that it almost becomes impossible to open eventually. It is also performed on post menopausal women as a final door closing.

It is also a possibility that this might even have roots in hunting and gathering times. If women were unable to have normal intercourse so easily then fewer babies would be born, leaving anal sex as the only 'safe sex' penetrative alternative. Being on the move meant a limit to how much each person could carry so they wouldn't have wanted several babies to lug about. But this is only my theory and is not provable.

Superstitions abound surrounding FGM, from thinking that if the clitoris isn't cut back it will keep growing and become a penis, to the belief that a woman is only pure and attractive once these parts of her anatomy are reduced or removed. Some even believe that the clitoris is dangerous to the man and physically coming into contact with it might kill him. These vastly imagined hysterical reactions to the female genitals are hard for many of us to understand. And although female libido can often be higher than a man's and women can, in theory, have sex repeatedly without needing a rest to become re-aroused, it still beggars belief that people have allowed this to effect them quite so drastically. Did our ancestors at some point decide the male libido could only remain a strong reflection of masculinity if the excessive female one was removed from the equation? It certainly seems as though this might be a part of the reason for FGM's to occur. It is well known that the female libido can make many men feel impotent. And it is also generally agreed that those with a higher libido are more likely to masturbate and/or be unfaithful in order to release it. In some cultures male masturbation is accepted while female masturbation is most definitely frowned upon.

The horror continues to grow with the discovery that the vast majority of these procedures are carried out by women on women without any anaesthetics, and often with non-sterile equipment or ritual knives. Being female this was gut wrenchingly difficult to read about. I can't get my head around how painful it must be and what on earth drives women to do this to each other.

The Temne people of Sierra Leone are one of many groups or tribes that still practice specific initiation ceremonies including FGM's. These rites of passage, once commonplace all over the world, only varied slightly in their physical expression. Temne tradition is rooted in the lunar cycle. The moon governs their lives and regulates pretty much every aspect. Although they acknowledge the sun, its relationship with them is not as intense or important. They have 12 months of roughly 29 days each and measure from new moon to full moon.

Each female in the tribe will at some point in her life go through Bondo, also known as Bundu, which lasts one year. This secret and entirely feminine preserve is kept shrouded in much mystery. So very little of what happens in a Bondo ritual is known about. The girl will be taken from her family, often to a wooded area, and undergo physical mutilation that in the past has varied from labial scratches to a full clitoral circumcision. Part of Bondo is meant to invoke the 'coming out' and is symbolic of the actual blood shedding that will occur during puberty. As already mentioned the circumcision is something we as Westerners find hard to accept or stomach; to us it is barbaric and unnecessary and in essence I'd agree. And as it limits the woman's ability to climax and means her levels of sexual arousal will be lessened, it certainly leads one to think this way. Regardless of the religious and cultural motivation, it is still upheld by modern day Temne. The evidence, no matter how unsavoury, is that it is very much the women who do it and keep it going as a traditional part of their lives. It is certainly believed among the Temne that a woman's sex drive is almost twice as high as a man's is. This might or might not have been seen as acceptable in ancient times but many modern day Temne seem to view it negatively.

The girls undergoing Bondo are kept hidden from the men especially and undergo other more magical and mysterious rituals and ceremonies closely guarded by other women. The release of an initiated Bondo woman back into her society is timed to coincide with when the other women consider she is at her most fertile. After Bondo the girl has her 'coming out' they hold a very unusual group celebration called 'e-lukne'. During 'e-lukne' the whole village cross-dress and dance and wave broken and worn out objects in the air. All ages participate and at the end any married Bondo woman may have sex with any man in the village if she wishes to. This aspect is particularly enjoyed by all concerned apparently. This letting down of hair is seen as 'transplanting' as gender exchanges and liberations are embraced with much enthusiasm. It must also follow that many babies are conceived at this time which makes me wonder just how important the actual parentage is to the Temne people. Maybe it is more important to keep the whole tribe happy with all the adhesion to traditional practises than to worry over who fathered

Menstruation and Birth

whose child. And as the women tend to do most of the child rearing then sharing the load is very much a part of normal daily life. The bond between the Bondo women is respected even more so than other tribal customs.

The men have a similar rite of passage for the boys called 'poro' but apparently it isn't in any way as long, drawn out and complicated as the women's Bondo rites. The Bondo women are joined in blood on all levels, even spiritually, and this sisterhood is formidable; even the chief of the tribe won't ever interfere with Bondo.

To people whose lives are lunar all is governed by the rise and fall of the moon. They have no less than eight names for the moon phases and Bondo occurs just before first quarter and just after last quarter. If we tally this up with harmonising the moon cycle to a woman's menstrual cycle we see that the first and last quarter tie up with the time of the ovum being released and the time of menses. The Temne say there are two periods of 'illness' for women each month — one is just post-ovulation and the other pre-menstrual. They see menses as represented by the dark of the moon and ovulation occurs when the moon is full. Most women who are sensitively tuned to their bodies would agree, these are the times of heightened emotions connected with the times of rising hormone levels. During the first half of the month there is a rise in oestrogen, and the second half of the month brings the height of progesterone. During the new moon, the whole village down tools. This is a day off and it is considered bad luck to work on this day.

This can tie up with other superstitions regarding the nature of the new moon energy. I was taught to avoid any magical work on the new moon as the energy was considered chaotic and potentially dangerous. Temne are not encouraged to greet any strangers on this day either. Sex is avoided during this time and the 'red' time is when women are, as in other tribal customs, isolated. Hunting is associated with the red phase and its associations might make one think this was so the men could escape a tribe of bleeding women. In theory this would stand up except for the fact that, in spite of synchrony, not all women of fertile age would be menstruating. Even with taking pregnancy and breast feeding out of the equation the Western concept of the monthly bleed is not always the case among tribal women. Amenorrhea or lack of menses can be due to many other factors including disease, over-exertion and malnutrition among other reasons. So the link is more likely to be purely bloody and no other.

This is just one of many cultural examples of FGM and its role in the society. With the Temne it seems an attempt to control female libido more than anything else. The fact that they have a free sex ceremony following it makes me think that at worst they only practice type one or two mutilation.

The age at which girls are put through this also varies from culture to culture. In Ethiopia it is done when the girls are only a few days old, whereas in Somalia the girls are often between 4-9 years old. But in some cultures it can continue up until fifteen years old. The fact that nearly all forms of FGM, regardless of culture, are carried out by women at the insistence of the girls is very hard for us to comprehend. In some cultures young girls will do it to themselves and then say a friend did it for her. The WHO is doing its best to re-educate people and lessen the numbers of women put through this but it is almost impossible to regulate. It is also estimated that up to 15% of the deaths that occur as a result of FGM's are never reported. I find it a very sad state of affairs and just as pointless as the majority of male circumcisions.

One reason for promoting both male and female circumcisions is hygiene. The belief that it is cleaner is promoted as a good enough reason in itself, but it seems to go hand in hand with the same argument currently in vogue for infantilizing women. For some reason in this so-called advanced 21st century world we also view female pubic hair with the same disdain. With the waxing and waning of cultural and cross cultural exchanges increasing, the constant desire to alter our genital appearance is unlikely to ever stop.

Birth

Birth is a messy, bloody business, so we are told, and for some this news is the most unpleasant factor to face. Yet it is rarely that bloody at all and what blood there is is life blood in its most splendid form. There is a little around the baby and some will seep from scratches or episiotomy wounds and the chord cutting moment but it is the placenta that is the bloodiest substance by far.

For any woman having a 'normal delivery' there will be blood, of that you can be sure, but the bulk of it is held in the after birth or placenta. This large, liver-like organ has nourished your unborn child from the earliest weeks of its development to the moment it emerges from the birth canal. In our modern Western world it is usually cast into a bucket and never seen again by the mother who pushed it from her womb.

Many superstitions surround the placenta and some advocate burying it in the earth for varying reasons. The Native American Navajo tribe believed in burying it to symbolically link the infant with the land and help its soul ground and connect with the tribe and environment it is born into. This practise of burying the placenta is common all over the world in tribal customs. The Lao of Kenya would bury the placenta of a girl infant on the left hand side of the house, as this is the side of vulnerability, while the male placenta was buried on the right corresponding with what they saw as the protective male side of the house. Thai culture would bury it under the birth tree of the infant. In Cambodia they also have an arboreal burial but this time there would be a spiky thorn tree or shrub planted over it to offer protection to the baby.

Ukrainian women often used the placenta to divine with, especially concerning any matters relating to health of the baby and the expected size of a woman's family. And up until relatively recently in South Africa it was customary to bury half of it and eat the other half, but under new health and safety food regulations it is now discouraged (though not enforced). There are also traditions in many cultures that have permeated to our shores for the consuming of the organ. But, apart from a few occasional requests, the vast majority of today's placentas find their way to the hospital incinerator. I do remember that during the 70s and 80s it resurfaced as a fashion, especially among feminists. Such women chose to take theirs home and cook it to access the goodness from it but think this might have been a passing phase and not one hugely embraced or encouraged by subsequent generations.

Cutting the chord has become extremely ritualistic these days and it is now fairly common for the husband to be offered the choice of symbolically releasing the baby from its mother into his waiting arms. I'm not too sure about this. Many men do indeed leap at the opportunity and it does amaze me how many are prepared to do it. Yet the maternal connection once excreted is quickly hidden away from view unless she or they choose to keep it and have asked in advance to do so. To allow the father a part in the birth is relatively new in society. Previously throughout our written history birth has been kept from the father as a mystery known only to women and the occasional male doctor or midwife. And when we consider that it is only in the last hundred years or so that we have had any form of officially recognised midwifery it is not surprising to know that previous to this it was the responsibility of female relatives and/or local shamans or witches.

The earliest school of midwifery was in Paris in the 1600s and the first person to write any official text on the subject was Louise Bourgoiuse (1563-1636). It then took until 1830 for Augustus Granville to start the first British Obstetrics Society in London and almost another 100 years before, in 1902, the Midwives Act made it law for midwives to be officially trained and midwifery to be recognised as a profession. Prior to these events, midwifery was kept in secret and often regarded as one of women's 'diseases'. Even in ancient Egypt, where medical operations and even cosmetic surgery was practised, apart from a few wall carvings depicting mothers with newly born children the art of midwifery was kept under wraps and no text remains of the practice.

It seems almost impossible to believe that millions of ancestors came into the world with little or no pain relief. This is thought to be because it was often considered an affront to God to offer any, and thereby release a woman from Eve's curse. Also, little or no real knowledge of what or how to deal with anything other than straightforward births was handed down. What little was, was often to wise women of the village or town who would be paid a small price for their essential services. It is no wonder that infant mortality was so high and death in childbirth considered normal and regrettably expected until quite recently in human history, though one can understand it in some part. No woman is as vulnerable as when she is in labour, her primal instincts urge her to hide and protect herself the best she can. Lacking this opportunity she will only want someone she trusts to be with her when she has her baby. For a first child it is especially frightening, so the fact that midwifery was left to mothers, aunts, older sisters and local 'witches' — and I use the term loosely — is not surprising. And for many women it was, and still is, a time when bleeding, especially after the birth, can be fatal.

To have a father deliberately play a part in birth was almost unheard of. Today, it is considered beneficial for fathers to have the option of watching their children come into the world should they wish to but I will also say that many men feel pressurised into this. For some men, being there to support their wives/partners as they go through the trials and tribulations of labour is wanted, but for others it is a terrifying thought; for a few, one they would rather not go through again. Speak to men about labour and several reactions occur. There are some who say watching and supporting the birth was and is the most beautiful treasured memory of their lives, while for others is was traumatic and uncomfortable as they felt helpless to aid the woman in any significant manner ,apart from being an object of venom for placing her in the situation in the first place.

For a few it is unbearable and they opt out, preferring to leave it to those who can cope. It is a matter of individual choice and I for one don't think for one minute that men should feel pressurised in any way to be witness if they don't wish to. It is far better to have sympathetic support, strength and empathy after all.

The blood of birth and the blood of menstruation are intertwined as one. Both are life sources and both are the most common forms of blood we are all going to encounter at some point in our lives. This magical elixir has been held in the grail as the ultimate difference between men and women eternally. As such, we should treat both as precious and sacred placing the placenta back where it belongs as a miracle of life. And unless there is a conflict between the mother's rhesus blood group and the baby's, the mixing of the two doesn't normally cause problems.

The bleeding after the birth varies from one woman to another and is comparable to a period but heavier. As the womb excretes the remains of the lining it contracts, giving the woman after birth pains similar but stronger than any regular menstrual cramps. But these contractions are clever for as the womb contracts back down, it stimulates the production of the milk for the baby and the red flow is exchanged for the white.

Post partum bleeding can be dangerous and knowing how to stem this bleed is also part of the experienced midwives skills. If a woman with such a bleed is allowed to go unchecked it can lead to death very quickly. There's a popular saying that is often misused and that is, 'only women bleed', not true of course but only women bleed quite so frequently and so much. With births lasting from a few minutes to hours to even a couple of days, it really can cause serious exhaustion, but for the vast majority it is fairly straightforward and therefore home births are currently experiencing a comeback. All women are different, some prefer the security a full medical environment gives them, whereas some see this artificial sterile place as alien to the natural process of birth.

Menopause

A subject that is often the butt of many a joke but rarely talked about sympathetically or sensibly is the menopause. Once a woman gets to roughly her mid to late forties, she is usually already displaying signs of what doctors describe as the peri-menopause. This lowering of hormones is marked in many ways but not all women are aware of, or have, actual symptoms.

Oestrogen levels drop, so the cycle can vary in length and heaviness of flow. Some women have lighter and lighter periods and some are the exact opposite, having heavier ones. Any normal pattern to them can go out of the window as periods develop a mind of their own. Very few women are lucky enough to just stop having them and that's that.

Going from being a fertile woman who sheds blood to an older more mature woman can be psychologically traumatic for some women, as well as having both a physical and emotional reaction. Suddenly finding yourself on the other side of the menopause is a strange place for most women to come to terms with. Knowing that her fertile days are over and that the rise and fall of hormones is never coming back is very strange for women who have spent most of their lives caught in the cycle. And simply having to acknowledge that no matter how much they want it their wombs have shut down for business is not always an easy one to reconcile, especially if a woman feel she has been cheated of children or not had as many as she'd liked. The physical changes alone can be disturbing and awkward. Their natural lubrication diminishes and sex can become uncomfortable unless aided with lubricants.

Some women experience a lowering of libido and some not so while some even say it increases. As the menopause sets in ,the progesterone levels also begin to drop off and periods can be missed, making many menopausal women panic that they could be pregnant. Hot flushes are common and described as an intense fire that comes from within and is impossible to escape from. Some sweat profusely with these and others not so. Either way they are uncomfortable and can be very embarrassing as well as inconvenient. Some women put on weight, some lose weight. Some become very confused and distracted, making concentration difficult. Short-term memory loss is also a common factor.

Many other negative side effects and diseases such as fibroids can happen at this age or earlier. Most women can expect to have come out the other side of this change by the time they are in their mid to late fifties — some earlier and some later, but these are the usual ranges. The menopause is not always understood and mood swings can be quite violent and dramatic, making normal PMT symptoms seem mild by comparison. There seem to be many things that all women can do to lessen the symptoms but often these are the things menopausal women are drawn to.

It is always advised by doctors and many health conscious people to stop smoking. This is all very well and might reduce some of the symptoms but as we all know, giving up can also send stress levels through the roof. Women are also advised to cut down alcohol significantly. Again, this is good advice but some women react in the opposite way and actually take up heavy drinking during their menopause as a way of dealing with the stress. Cutting down caffeine is another one on the hit list; it does indeed increase the chances of hot flushes. Eating sensibly but allowing for carbohydrate cravings (they raise serotonin levels and can help, in moderation) is often cited. Taking regular exercise is encouraged, but then it is common sense if possible. Many doctors and health advisers will also say you should continue to enjoy a sex life if possible. This is all very well if possible but many women find sex goes off the menu for a few years. Either ingesting or applying yam in cream form on the lower stomach and breasts to maintain progesterone levels helps. Taking natural plant oestrogens or asking for an oestrogen cream, as some modern menopausal creams contain both hormones, can be helpful also. And finally if all else fails, ask the doctor about HRT or the coil implant. All of these things can help but aren't always easy to stick to.

The sheer number of women experiencing menopause has grown considerably over the last hundred years or so. We are living far longer than many of our ancestors and in greater numbers. Never before in our history have there been so many women having regular monthly bleeds and living long enough to experience the menopause. With increased numbers, good health, longer lives and less pregnancies, menstruation and menopause have become big business. With literally billions being spent on sanitary wear and HRT each year, it costs a fortune to be female in the developed world. And it doesn't seem necessarily any better to be born to an indigenous native village if FGM is anything to go by. If women are cursed I would say it is both by fear and prejudice surrounding their mysteries and the rising cost of supressing and hiding them from the outside world.

Goddess Ritual to invoke Hekate

The first chapter presents a triple problem in so much as it represents all three of the female cycles and, due to the emphasis being on blood rituals, that element needs to be included. After some consideration I decided to go with Hekate as she is a Moon deity and a triple-faced Goddess and has associations with sex and blood. There are some who would consider her appropriate and others less so. Being a Greek Goddess associated with the underworld, crossroads, prophecy and witchcraft she is often seen as the patron of witches past and present.

Although not normally seen as a fertility Goddess as such, she still embodies the darkness or void from which new life can spring forth. To me she has all three aspects pretty well covered. As maid, she is budding and becoming fertile; as mother she is in the bloom of her fertile phase; as crone she covers the post-menopausal period of our lives. To me she has all three aspects pretty well covered, although it is more than likely that her original form from south-west Anatolia was as a singularly presented force. The 'Holy Trinity' aspect is a later import, possibly from Egypt, although there we have the Father, mother, and son represented.

This is not a Goddess to experiment with. Often seen as the Queen of the infernal realms, she deals with the hidden side of our psyche and the buried knowledge we all need to remember. She has an incredibly powerful force that is thundering in its manifestation. Having Hekate arrive in a ritual is akin to a massive earthquake occurring. She can sometimes try and take possession, which might be perilous to a non initiate on her path or one who is not accustomed to one like her. Rituals to Hekate can be done either in solitary capacity or in a group or coven. The best time to call on Hekate is during the dark of the moon. The darkness of the womb and moon resonate well together.

Black is a colour associated with her but people often use three candles one red, one white and one black for each of her aspects.

Menstruation and Birth

Keys, ropes and athames are also linked with her and many people like to have a representation of the three way crossroads present. This can be done in salt on the altar cloth or drawn on paper.

Normal offerings of wine or beer and food etc. should also be present. Hekate likes nuts, particularly almonds, herbs such as tarragon and fennel, wine, beer and cider.

A spare sterile blade or needle for offering your blood is useful unless you plan to give of your menstrual blood which is also appreciated by Hekate. Black stones such as obsidian, jet and onyx are good, as are images of black dogs.

Circle casting is optional. My own personal feeling is that the deity herself can protect you from harm, but invoking the Cerberus or three-headed wolf is quite sufficient for protection of perimeter.

Calling the quarters is different from the right-hand path (RHP). Instead of merely asking the 'spirits' of each direction to be present, with Hekate it is a triangle so three directions are summoned. I advocate Lucifer in the East, Lilith in the South and Samael in the West.

This is only a minute fraction of the witch magic of Hekate. Should you wish to explore further then studying the Qliphoth or hidden side of the Tree of Life is advised.

Maid Calling — If planning fertility, calling Hekate will answer to your sexual energy. You can give blood as well but it isn't essential. If wanting help with periods then offer menstrual blood. This can be easily caught in a 'mooncup' (eco-friendly cups used instead of pads or tampons). Sprinkle the blood on and in both the food and liquor offering.

Mother — If asking for help protecting an unborn child and help during childbirth or with the actual childbirth it is best to procure blood from both parents. This can be added to the burning incense.

Menopause/post menopause — If wanting help crossing this final menstrual stage of life Hekate can aid your crossing. Providing you are still bleeding each month then offer up some menstrual blood. If your periods have stopped then offer her normal blood. Place it in an upturned walnut shell.

All blood offerings need burying at a T shaped or three way crossroads after ritual to ground and earth your ritual.

She originates from ancient Anatolia, modern day Turkey. Her main centre was Lagina and then she gained popularity in Athens. Most temple based rituals would be for a specific festival or purpose and include offerings, often blood related, dancing, music and possibly sex. Many modern day devotees to her still like to give offerings and often include sex.

A well respected expert on Hekate from a neo-pagan perspective is Mark Alan Smith and his book Queen of Hell has become hugely popular among those who work with Hekate.

Her sigil is usually a trident.

The structure and format of the ritual depends on each person's tradition and or coven.

The Calling

I call upon the Goddess Hekate

The mistress of the crossroads ………..She who aids our crossing points

The Queen of the witches……….She who weaves the magical forces within and without

The mother of the Angels……She who created the messengers between the gods and man

The keeper of arcane knowledge…….She who knows all there ever has been or ever will be

The key holder of the gates to the mysteries of the underworld and the necromancer supreme….She who traverses death and dances with its shadow

Menstruation and Birth

Hear me/us as I/we call upon you to make your presence felt here in this sacred space made so in your honour this witching hour on this dark moon night.

Oh most mighty and powerful terrifying lady, she who is three in one, who is maid, mother and crone, aid us in our quest tonight.

Hear me/us as I/we call upon you to rise from the void and travel the infinite distance to cross the veil and make manifest your energy on this plane for us tonight.

We are but blind children in your presence, forgive us our ignorance, protect us from any harm your energy might cause, and be patient with us as we reach to touch the hem of your skirts.

Hail Hekate the most ancient, the wise, the maid, the mother and the crone!

We beg you accept our humble offerings, accept our gratitude for gifts already bestowed upon us. We ask that you listen to our prayers and answer our deepest wishes made here in your name tonight.

Hail Hekate, the one before time, the one from the east who travelled west!

She who loves the moon light and is all that is darkness and not understood

She who lacks a consort for the cosmos itself is her family

She who rose from primordial times and created all that came before and all that is to come, we await your presence with open minds, open hearts and our bodies prepared for your arrival.

Hail Hekate!!

Hail Hekate!!

Hail Hekate!!

(Communion — the raising of sexual energy, either auto-erotic or with another, she likes unbridled lust and answers best to this).

Oh mother of mysteries whose image was sent to us from an ancient time and place before history was recorded I/we give our most heartfelt thanks to you for gracing us with your infernal presence here this dark moon night.

We are wiser for your coming forth by night
We are energised by your power from within to without
We are made magical to manifest our dreams and learn from our nightmares
All in your name Hekate
We bid ye farewell.

CHAPTER TWO
Hunting

Views regarding when hominoids began hunting are constantly changing with each new discovery. It has been generally accepted that we began as scavengers and foragers relying on what we could find easily in whatever environment we happened to be in. But at some point we began to hunt. Whether we started out as fishermen initially is not known for sure. The 'Out of Africa' theory that is currently being challenged by new findings about our evolution and migration always presumed we followed the shoreline. This would mean we were probably fishermen. But the advent of tool making and mastery of fire was our turning point and the beginning of what would accelerate our evolution. Even homo-erectus has provided evidence of rudimentary tools, and fires being lit deliberately. This would date hunting to over 1.5 million years old.

The proceeds of the hunt seem to have provided our ancestors with the complex proteins necessary for modern homo-sapiens to develop such large brains. To hunt an animal for food requires skill. Knowledge regarding the habits and nature of the prey has to be acquired. Efficient tools, weapons or traps have to be made or set. It might well be that some of the earliest hunting took the style of families utilising fire as a means to chase and direct animals in a direction of their choice, such as over a cliff for example. The creation of flint and obsidian spears, and axe heads to kill prey takes great skill and very few people could manage that today if they had to. It takes a surprising amount of patience and skill to become a flint knapper.

From the fossil record and other archaeological finds it seems we have always been omnivores. Even our closest primate relative the chimpanzee is an omnivore. Modern humans have been in their current anatomical form for at least 200,000 years and it seems that the vast majority of that has been spent eating a diverse diet. It is only over the last 8-12,000 years that we have been farming and domesticating animals. So it would transpire that the vast majority of our pre-history was spent scavenging and hunting for food. Scavenging in itself is an art that leads to tracking and gradually learning about the habits of the animals in your environment.

This ability that mankind developed to hunt and kill food is at the very core of our nature and a true reflection of our place in the animal kingdom. We may have begun as chimpanzees but even chimps are omnivores. It is partly due to our ability to survive on such a variety of foodstuffs that we have arrived at the point we are today in this sophisticated world of culinary cuisine. Yet once upon a time, not so long ago, we all depended on the hunt.

It is believed that our very earliest form of meat eating was scavenging on dead carcasses. This would have occurred way before modern homo-sapiens evolved, around the time of homo-erectus. But it is also believed by many modern palaeo-anthropologists that by eating the bone marrow and meat of beasts, we accelerated our brain development and through this became more intelligent and cognitive as a result. If we hadn't begun eating meat, we might still be swinging from the trees and never have stood upright.

Hunting

Current thinking among archaeologists and anthropologists is that we stood up in order to move faster and be able to carry things. Darwin proposed that it was due to the need to free the hands for tool making but apes and chimps do this sort of thing and still remain mostly on all fours. Carol Ward is an associate professor in the department of anthropology and the department of pathology and anatomical sciences at the University of Missouri at Columbia and she thinks it most likely that we were developing more sophisticated survival methods, including carrying tools and weapons and small amounts of foodstuffs. This ability would give us an edge over the absolute necessity to have a successful hunt or scavenge each day. If we were able to retain the tools and carry them from place to place, it cut down the time and energy required to create new ones. The value placed upon early tools and weapons must have been very high.

By comparing the dietary requirements between apes and humans, it is fairly obvious that we became the bigger meat eaters. Chimps and apes might only procure 6-8% of their proteins from animal sources, whereas modern humans obtain up to 22% from meat. Our ability to stand up has much to do with hunting, or the emergence of it, alongside the changes in resources our ancestors found as they migrated from one place to another.

As a large ape, we lack efficient hunting tools. Our teeth are not particularly dangerous and nor are our nails. As a hunting machine, the human body is a failure apart from two massive differences: our brains and our opposable thumbs. Our ability to make crude rudimentary tools to break into bones to get at marrow in dead carcasses was the beginning of what would eventually lead to the creation of the microchip. But it all began with our earliest ancestors and their desire to get at the nutrients hidden inside seemingly difficult nooks and crannies.

For modern homo-sapiens, the climate has changed on a frequent basis. In the time mankind has been on the planet he has already survived serious global natural catastrophes and has overcome nearly all of the obstacles placed in his way. And as we overcame, so our lust for blood and flesh grew. Earliest hunting tools were made of bone, wood, stone etc. and were often very finely crafted. Even one simple arrowhead made of flint could take hours to refine and the detail of some is extraordinary. The variety of arrowheads and spearheads is also amazing. Each one seemed crafted for a very specific task. Some were for throwing or firing from a bow and some for direct close interaction with the intended kill. This proves how important each tool was. The amount of time invested in making it meant it became invaluable to the person who owned it.

Our whole human history has been built on the back of hunting and yet not all people are hunters. Hunters seem to be of a particular type of personality. Killing does not come naturally to everyone. The vast majority of people prefer not to kill their own dinner, and our ancestors were probably no different in this. There were some that were better at gathering and scavenging and some that were good at killing. It is good news for many vegans and vegetarians, no doubt, that it doesn't seem to be in everyone's nature to get blooded.

It is ridiculous to imagine that pre-historic man hunted to feed a bloodlust. His most basic need was way more fundamental and was that of securing regular food source. But out of these needs came rituals and superstitions and otherworldly journeys. We might not ever know what in our cognitive thought processes gave birth to shamanism. It might have been to do with hunting but could be more specifically linked with death. Whether this was death of those we loved or animals we killed is not known. It is the earliest form of human spiritual expression that we know of. So whether it was the death of a person in a tribe or clan, or the death of the hunt, the need to still acknowledge the spirit of the ancestor or animal seems very important indeed.

Hunting

Shamanism and animism are often part of each other and they both seem to stem from a very early form of belief. To some it is the belief that everything has spirit, even mountains, rivers, trees etc. This belief in animism is found all over the world seemingly having evolved along very closely related paths among groups of people that had never met. It seems part of our collective evolution to have trodden this road. Blood in itself isn't always seen as especially important in every indigenous group but it is more so in some than others. And the one place it is always found and interacted with is the hunt.

The primary function of hunting was to kill animals for food. The blood was incidental yet also provided a direct link between ourselves and the animal kingdom. It is entirely feasible to imagine that our ancestors of 200,000 years ago viewed the animal kingdom in a slightly different way to us. Not only did they see themselves as animals and an integral part of the greater environment but they would have probably graded animals into groups. The three I feel were of most relevance to a hunter were; their prey, the predators and the mysterious/poisonous. One group is edible, one might eat us and one is best left alone, which seems all quite simple really. And until we started working with or using animals for hunting and/or carrying us this most probably remained the same. But many animals have similar physical characteristics to man and also bleed just as we do and have birth and death cycles just as we have.

As the relationships we had with each group grew, greater respect for them also evolved and gave birth to the elaborate cave drawings and other associated art form the prehistoric era. With the prey group the relationship became dependent and therefore more complex and deeper as a consequence. It also seems possible that our most ancient of hunting ancestors also began to feel that they became the animals that they ate. Our food source became us and we them. With beliefs such as the blood containing the life source and the spiritual home of a person or animal growing ,so our relationships intensified.

Respect and reverence was given to many predators, such as lions and crocodiles and other creatures, with some cultures choosing to avoid them and others elevating them to God and Goddess status. But there are just as many, if not more, images of the ones we ate than any other group. The blood was revered and the most common tradition that has survived until present day was that of 'being blooded'. Being blooded takes various forms depending on minor differences between groups or tribes of people that hunt. This practise usually comprises of initiates to the hunt being smeared with the blood of their first kill.

The 'Blooding Rite', common to parts of Western Europe and America appears to have been spawned by the veneration of St Hubert. Hubert lived in the Ardennes in France around 650AD. It is said that he lost his wife during childbirth and his reaction was to withdraw from his courtly duties. He went to the forest in Ardennes. Here he spent his time hunting and this became his only passion. He was a hunter of deer mostly but boar also and rode on horse back hunting with hounds.

The story goes that on a Good Friday morning he went hunting as normal and found a magnificent stag to pursue. To his amazement at one point the stag suddenly turned towards him and stopped in its tracks. Hubert saw a golden glowing crucifix appear between the stag's antlers and a voice emanated from the beast. It said; *"Hubert, unless thou turnest to the Lord, and leadest an holy life, thou shalt quickly go down into hell"*. Hubert got off his horse and fell to his knees saying, "Lord, what wouldst Thou have me do?" He received the answer, *"Go and seek Lambert, and he will instruct you."* He is then said to have gone to Bishop Lambert, who took him on as a potential cleric. Hubert rose through the priestly ranks quite quickly, having handed his lordly title over to his brother, sold all his worldly goods and distributed his wealth among the poor. He was elevated to sainthood as a result of his vision and lifetime dedication to Holy work. St Hubert of Liège is patron of metalworkers, huntsmen and dogs, among a few other things besides. It is said that this story was first told as the legend of St Eustace or Placidus. It was first attributed to St Hubert in the 15th century. In honour of St Hubert, hunters will smear themselves on the face with the blood of their fresh kill. And so this essentially Roman tradition was reborn with St Hubert and is still to this day practiced among hunters throughout Europe and North America.

Although many modern hunters view this with amusement as some sort of vague historical religious ritual that should probably be relegated to the mists of time, this tradition carried on in this country until relatively recently. Former British fox hunts still blooded their new members at the site of their first witnessed kill until the practise was banned a few years ago. I can remember working in a riding school that had a pony club attached to it and would see young children return from a days hunting with faces reddened in fox blood. Although I still consider fox hunting unnecessary, it was not without its peculiar fascinations.

Some advocate eating the still-beating heart as a sign of respect for the creature killed, thinking that in doing this the person concerned would take on the spirit of the dead animal. The theory then being that the hunter who ate the heart of a deer, for example, would become the animal, if he wished, at a later date during trance, ritual or sweat lodge journeys. This would increase their connection with the beast and any deity connected with it.

Many of a pagan persuasion today will hold both pre hunt and post-hunt rituals to deities and ancestral hunters. They believe that this will aid them in the hunt, give them spiritual absolution and permission to kill an animal whilst increase their sensitivities, enabling them to be more attuned hunters. It also increases their devotion and spiritual respect for the animal.

It is also believed among many who do hunt for food to this day that this blooding practice evolved from a more incredible past. Modern paleo-anthropologists say that the parts of the body first consumed were the organs, so offal and brain and marrow were the initial ports of call to a hungry tribe surrounding its kill. This makes sense for many reasons. One is that, with the exception of marrow, these soft tissues were the easiest to eat straight away. They also contain high levels of fat and proteins and they don't store as well as muscle. And a still-beating heart also contains another highly prized substance, adrenaline. To consume adrenaline is one of nature's instant highs, comparable to amphetamines, and the drinking of blood was, and still is in some cultures, a highly valued practice. This would have been highly sought after and may well be the reason alpha males and females emerged. The race to be the best hunter and get to the kill first to extract the adrenaline would have been great. The early hunting men and women could be today's modern extreme sport junkies. Hunting, like sport, sex and pain releases endorphins and adrenalin. This is a potent enough mixture when self-produced but if you add the adrenaline of a fresh kill into it you get an even bigger high. This would be very addictive

And so as those who hunted developed these blood traditions and rituals, they became more and more sophisticated in their tools and skills. But early hunters didn't discriminate, they had to learn the hard way, and although they achieved great successes in mastering hunting and killing they were often too successful.

A tradition attached to some Native American tribes and hunters on mainland Europe is the one of the last bite. With Native Americans, it became tradition to place a corn cob in the mouth of the fresh kill. This was a mark of respect to the animal and gave it a symbolic last meal. This tradition might well have been an import from Mainland Europe as there is much evidence in countries such as Germany that a similar tradition known as the 'branch sign' is still used to this day. In German it is called the 'lesser bissen' or last bite. A sprig or small branch of pine is placed in the mouth of the fresh kill and then placed in the left hand side of the hunters cap. It is normally presented after a hunter has killed his first cloven animal. The branch is worn until sunset of that day. Another form of 'branch sign' was the placing of sprigs or branches in the earth to convey messages to other members of the hunt. During a hunt, hunters can sprawl out over a large area and in places such as woodland where visibility is less these branch signs were invaluable. This practise grew and versions of it were incorporated into military and scouting usage throughout most countries.

It also seems that mankind generally became too proficient at hunting. Occasionally he over hunted and almost drove himself to the brink of starvation being left with cannibalism as his only option before realising that hunting, like breeding, needed to be more selective. And so he learnt to watch and study his prey with keen observation. He made an in-depth study of the animals he sought and he developed many spiritual beliefs and shamanic practises around these hunts. By learning their breeding cycles and following the herds, he knew which beasts to hunt and when best to hunt them. Tracking became his most important skill to master. He needed to know how to recognise the habits, foot marks, scents and excretions of his prey and how to stay downwind of it. He also mastered trapping, which became an even easier method of hunting and far less tiring. Our most primitive brain will always lead us to the easiest way to do things as this uses less energy. Why waste more energy on hunting than you will get from the kill? Trapping requires people to be at least semi-settled for a while. It might take a few hours or a few days to trap an animal. Hunting and trapping might have co-evolved but they are very different and trapping doesn't seem to have any blood rite or ritual associated with it. It seems that hunting has the stronger spiritual aspect to it.

It is not often realised just how much our Neolithic ancestors changed their environment in order to survive. Neolithic man set fire to huge areas of land to clear trees, encouraging grass to grow knowing that it would attract grazing beasts long before he began farming the land. In this country early blood would have been found in deer, boar, hares, sheep and goats among others. It is also more common for us to eat herbivores than carnivores. Some say this is due to the fact that most carnivores had efficient teeth and claws to fight back with or it could be that we prefer the taste of herbivores. But I think it is a numbers game. The numbers of herbivores far outweighs the number of carnivores, so they were and still are more prolific. Grazing herds are just that, herds. There is a higher likelihood of success in catching one from many than one of one. Our ancestors played the odds and won. And although fishing would have also occurred, as it still does, it wasn't quite the same as hunting and doesn't seem to have the ritualistic trademarks of bloodlust. Indeed to this day fishing is considered as an altogether separate activity from hunting land beasts.

From their emergence in Africa to the Middle Eastern Fertile Crescent it took modern homo-sapiens roughly 40,000 years to begin farming, an activity that only evolved about 8-10,000 years ago. Prior to this, from evidence we currently have, it seems that they were exclusively hunters and gatherers. During this time our earliest religious and spiritual beliefs were formed and blood had much to do with them. From the most ancient of cave paintings we see people hunting with spears and bows for cloven beasts, birds and smaller animals. Here men and women work together in mutual co-operation to outwit and out manoeuvre the animals they hunted. And it follows that a great and detailed study of the desired prey would grow over time and hunting would become less reliant on opportune moments and more about pre-planning and preparation. Considering the wide variety of flint arrows and spearheads found it is evident that this was so. And so with such variety of weapons to hunt with, man took another massive leap in his survival history: he began to pick and choose his meals.

The more dependent they became on specific beasts, the more they sought to know and — if possible — direct and control them. The blood of the kill may have begun as a secondary gain but the essence of life in the hunt was strong and the desire to partake of it was laced with lust for the red stuff. Only those who have taken part in hunting can appreciate the excitement generated. This bloodlust did mature into a mere saying but for those who still hunt on foot or horse it is a powerful primal force that connects them directly with their ancestors and the feelings around the hunt for blood.

As the animal is sighted, a surge of adrenaline is produced urging you on towards it. As the animal takes flight, more adrenaline is pumped through the system, and as you exert energy to take chase after it, endorphins are kicking in giving you a natural high. This positive association derives from the most primitive source of all, that of survival and eating. Eating also releases happy hormones into our blood streams and so hunting and eating the kill are potent driving forces in themselves, but when you add the desire to be first and get the greater high and even more positive association into the equation, you can understand that even from a purely physiological point of view, hunting is bloody and addictive stuff!

Sami Bear Ritual

The various peoples of the far northern hemisphere share a common reverence for bears. The Sami of northernmost Norway, Sweden and Finland were no exception. Bears have a supernatural mystery surrounding them and are very much an apex predator on a par, if not above us. Common elements in bear ceremonies between tribes on different continents have intrigued anthropologists. One shared similarity is the belief that the bear is a gatekeeper to the mystical or supernatural world.

When we look at the geography of the northern hemisphere it is not so surprising. At some points in our shared human history this massive area became one frozen land mass. And it is not stretching our imaginations too far to see how Native Americans, Europeans and Eurasians might once have literally met sharing common links and experiences and beliefs, From these groups, such as the Sami, Gilyaks, Tungus and Native American tribes, a bear cult could have developed.

Various unsubstantiated but interesting theories have been proposed for why these similarities have developed. The bear is an apex hunter; he is king of his domain. He can, like man, hunt on land or in lakes, rivers and oceans. He can stand on two legs if needs be and he also poses a direct threat to man and easily kills us if he needs to. But he isn't a natural predator of man. Like a lion, he doesn't see the need to kill us unless we pose a threat to him. We are most definitely not on their preferred diet list. Most fellow apex predators leave each other alone for the most part. And so the bear is held in very high esteem. The bear might be seen as the living spirit of an ancestor, thereby gaining a direct link with the other world or world of the dead. The bear is a very high ranking deity in tribes that live among them and from this elevation and mutual respect came beliefs that in order to have a successful days hunting or fishing the spirit of the bear must be appeased and pleased. It is also believed that our ancestors felt guilt connected with having to kill a bear or any animal they held in high regard and had developed divine or Godly reverence for.

The Sami predominantly hunted reindeer and fished. This placed them on the same hunting level as the bear; we shared the same dinner. So whereever herds of reindeer were bears were also often found. And the same can be said for fishing. The Sami, the Native Americans in the far north and the Siberian peoples all saw the bear as sacred. Comparable folk wisdoms developed surrounding not only bears but all other aspects of the shared environment.

Hunting

The Sami had a very particular order of events surrounding the bear hunt. It always took place during the hibernation season with bears being literally awoken and taken from their dens whilst at their sleepiest. A shaman known as a Noajdde or drummer would be consulted before the hunt left for the bear's den. The Noajdde would also accompany them and choose the hunter to kill the bear. The bear is killed by a spear or lance that has a brass ring attached to it. This was more to annoy and aggravate the bear into coming out of its den, whereupon the other hunters would attack it with various weapons. The freshly killed bear would then be struck with twigs and birch brash. A ring of soft birch would be put around the bear's lower jaw. The primary bear hunter (the one with the brass ring) would tie this to his waist and tug at it whilst singing a specific song to mean he has become the bear's master.

Once the hunt returns to the village with their kill they are greeted by women who spit elder bark juice at their faces. The one with the ring goes to his home and knocks three times before being allowed in. The brass ring is kept wrapped up until after the bear ceremonial meal. Women were not allowed to cook or prepare the bear meat and had to keep their heads covered for up to five days after the ceremony. Another weird aspect is that they could only look at the primary bear killer through a brass ring.

After three days, the bear skin is stretched out and offerings made to its spirit and lain upon the skin. After feasting the ring is removed and the women and children attach a chain to it that they tie to the bear's tail. The ring and bones of the bear are buried by men and the skin is lain out and shot at to prevent the spirit of the bear killing any of the women and children of the village.

It is interesting to me as someone who lives in East Anglia in the UK that we have an area known as the Fens. The Sami were sometimes called Lapp or Fenn. Evidence that reindeer hunting once occurred as far north as Staffordshire in this country exists.

and the Fens is an area that was once a mixture of marshland and islands of drier land that people could set up temporary camps on. We have always had waves of Scandinavian influences arriving on our shores and their mystical and magical practices do bare strong similarities with Sami shamanism.

The Ainu and Gilyak peoples also had very similar bear hunting ceremonies. They too viewed the bear as the mediator between the people and the spirit of the forest. The Gilyak peoples of Siberia would capture a bear cub in spring. They would also kill the mother if needed, but it was the cub they wanted. They would keep it and feed it and honour it for several months and then kill it in an elaborate ceremony ending with the bear being shot by an arrow. Its head and skin were laid out facing west and symbolic offerings made to its mouth. Only the elder men of the village were allowed to look after and kill the bear. Throughout its time with the people it was treated well and prayers offered up to its spirit to think well of them.

The Ainu of northern Japan also capture a bear cub in the spring. It is looked after for up to 18 months by villagers. The festival during which the bear is killed is called the Lymante festival and it takes place during September or October. The bear is shot with arrows and then strangled whilst women wail and cry at its death. Elder men skin the bear and, like the Sami and the Gilyak, they leave the head attached to the skin and lay it out on an altar and offer it food and sake whilst praying to the Goddess of fire. The liver is cut into small pieces and eaten straight away and men drink its blood in small cups. The meat is eaten on the next day.

Maasai Lion Hunt

The Maasai of African savannahs have a lion hunting rite of passage for young warriors. It used to be that a young man would hunt a male lion alone. This would enable him to prove his courage, strength and ability to fight men if the need arose. These days, because of lower lion numbers and a desire by the Maasai to allow lion numbers to increase again they are encouraged to do this in groups. They always avoid sick or diseased lions and females. It is only considered brave to hunt down and kill an adult male lion.

There is much secrecy surrounding this hunt. The men plan it and arrange the details and time and place without the knowledge spreading to the rest of the tribe. Once they are ready to leave, they do it just before dawn so as not to disturb anyone in the tribe or village that might stop them. They don't eat the meat of the lion but do take the claws, mane and tail to adorn themselves with on special ceremonial celebrations.

A warrior is expected to hunt lions every 10-15 adult years and keep a count of the lions he has killed. This may seem unethical to us in the west and is illegal in protected reserves but this is an ancient tradition and one they still maintain. Sometimes lions are killed in revenge attacks for the loss of domesticated cattle and sheep and goats to lions. It is an uneasy relationship and always has been.

Young warriors are known as Ilbarnot and the older warriors are the Ilmorijo who decide all the finer details of the hunt. The hunt itself involves tracking and following signs such as vulture activity which might indicate a lion kill. The choice of which Ilbarnot can hunt lions is a battle in itself. Often older warriors will argue over which young men are worthy of the hunt and the young men will jostle and fight with the older ones to prove themselves brave and strong enough. The success of the hunt initiates a week long celebration. Whoever speared the lion first receives a beaded ceremonial strap to wear.

Surprisingly hunting an adult male lion is not easy. Lions avoid us if they can. They have much sense. So they are often tracked for up to ten hours and then chased and deliberately wound up and irritated by threatening to take its kill or pursuing it with rattles and bells to provoke anger in the beast and bring on an attack.

After the meat ceremony, when a warrior becomes a junior elder, he must throw the lion mane away. But first he must sacrifice a sheep and grease the lion mane with its oils mixed with ochre. At this time, the warrior must slaughter a sheep and grease the mane with a mixture of sheep oil and ochre. He is seen as honouring the spirit of the lion by doing this.

The lion tail is sent to women to add beads to, before being returned to the warrior who wins a wrestling fight with other warriors. The warriors will look after and keep safe the lion's tail in their manyatta (warriors camp), until he retires from warriorhood. The tail is thrown away after a ceremony known as Enuoto.

This example of hunting purely for a rite of passage and not consuming the animal is not as common as ones that include eating the meat afterwards. We often look back on big game hunting colonialists with horror, and with good reason. But it is easy to see how they viewed the hunt in a similar manner. These days hunting to cull numbers is common and we do it with a large variety of animals. Any that seem to be outgrowing resources, threatening our own, or carrying diseases are seen as fair game to cull. Vermin come under this banner, and most culls take place when animals are not in the breeding season. Game birds and deer are still hunted legally in this country. Fox hunting has now been outlawed but gamekeepers are allowed to trap them and shoot them. I'm never too sure which is worse.

The blood of the hunt still beats in many people today. They may not realise all the reasons for their desires, or why they wish to get up close and personal to death but at a deep and primal level it is most probably an ancestral bloodlust that spurs them on. The animals they hunted provided food, their skins provided clothing and shelter, the bones became tools and all of the animal was utilised. If one had to define a smell to sum up the hunting and gathering period in human history it would be blood, which has an aroma akin to copper. And if you were that ancestor sitting in your rudimentary wood and skin shelter, wearing furs and eating meat from a fresh kill, this would be all you could smell. That in itself evokes nostalgic ancestral memories that we all share and have in common but for the most part are completely unaware of in this modern, chemical-based, technological era of humanity. Yet as our present lifestyles seem unsustainable it might pay for all of us to re-connect with our more primitive past and learn to see blood in a much more positive light before we detach too far from it and are unable to hunt ever again.

Man Hunting Man

'There is no hunting like the hunting of man, and those who have hunted armed men long enough and liked it, never care for anything else thereafter.' Ernest Hemingway.

It would be easy to think this came under the simple label of war but the type of hunting I am looking at here is rarer. This is the deliberate tracking down and hunting of individual men by another man or men. Whether it is for sport or to exact out a perceived punishment or some sick and twisted game played out by an equally perverted mind, it is different to the art of the warrior.

The most common example that is perfectly legal in the vast majority of countries is police work. Often police or law enforcers will have to hunt down men and women to bring them to justice. This type of detective work is accepted by societies, by and large. Bounty hunters probably come a close second.

The film industry has often been inspired by this concept and many a film has been spawned by it. Predator films for example. But in reality it is quite rare. People might have personal vendettas against others and choose to take the law into their own hands and become vigilantes, but to actually hunt down a person with the sole aim of killing them doesn't happen too often. And to kidnap a person purely to set them free and then pursue them is even rarer.

But in essence we have all done this. The children's game of 'tag' or 'it' or 'chase' etc. is just that, albeit in a very tame way, as it is carried out in parks and gardens and school playgrounds. 'Hide and seek' is another example that we have all gained a buzz from at some point in our lives. But it seems the primal urge to chase is within us all and although it probably does stem from a desire to hunt our food it can easily spill over into hunting purely for fun.

As with most of the chapters, I've included a ritual to a pagan deity/entity connected to the subject matter of the chapter in mind and this one is to the Celtic/Germanic God Cernunnos.

Hunting

Ritual to invoke Cernunnos

Very little is actually known through archaeology about Cernunnos. His name has been discovered twice. One is on the inside of the famous Gundestrap Cauldron that was found in the village of the same name in the parish of Aars in Himmerland Denmark. It is thought to have been made at some point between 200BCE to 300AD Made of mostly silver with gold gilt it was obviously an expensive item once belonging to a rich person or tribe. His appearance in it almost looks as if it might be at home in India. Sitting in a lotus position, we have a horned God with the antlers of a deer. He holds a mythical ram headed snake in his left hand and a gold torc in his right. He is surrounded by beasts including a deer, boar, cat, fox and others besides. Modern pagans often depict him with an erection to symbolise his link with male sexuality. As the preceding chapter has been all about hunting it felt instinctively right to have an example of a Cernunnos ritual for people to consider, or use as they see fit.

He is also seen up high on the Pillar of the Boatman. This massive pillar was erected by the Romans and placed in a temple by the Seine in what is now France and what was then Gaul. The pillar was a dedicated gift in honour of Tiberius Caeser Augustus that was commissioned by the guild of sailors in Lutetia or what is now Paris. This is the only ancient artefact to date that has been discovered that actually calls him Cernunnos. His inclusion appears to be of high status and an attempt to appease his followers and to recognise him as they went conquering their way through what they saw as his kingdom.

There are many differing opinions as to the meanings of his imagery. The torc was an object that only the richest tribal leaders could afford. It might represent the proceeds of the hunt and seems to be saying that he can aid you in hunting and gaining profits from it. So he is often associated with wealth. It is mainly through comparing other similar Celtic imagery that modern day archaeologists and historians are able to piece together the most likely reason for such symbolism.

The ram-headed snake however confuses most. Rams are creatures known for rushing headlong at people and butting them. Snakes can be taken by surprise and strike at us if we disturb or provoke them, accidently or not. Both creatures are very instinctive and can cause much harm. The Druids might have had a secret knowledge or message attached to this image but left precious few clues. We can only surmise its meaning. To me he seems to be saying that true wealth is not mastery of nature and acquisition of material goods, but being like him, at one with and at peace with nature. And in most cults the snake represents rejuvenation, re-birth and the activation of primal kundalini. His peaceful seated position surrounded by the beasts of the hunt also seems to be saying that he holds dominion over the wilder aspects and can be called upon both to aid you in your hunting and also protect you from any potential harm.

This ritual is best done outside and preferably in woodland.

The time of day doesn't seem overly important to me. Our 'out of Africa' ancestors probably did most of their hunting around mid day; the evidence seems to lean towards us taking advantage of the time when many animals are sleepy. But ancestors from the northern hemisphere might well have also hunted during full moons at night.

You will need a symbolic hunting weapon; this can be anything from a spear, to a knife, to a sharpened flint.

You will need an offering to give him. In the case of this book it is merely a few drops of your own blood or that of a freshly killed animal, like a rabbit for example, that you have hunted and killed yourself. If not wishing to become the literal hunter then your own blood is fine. And if neither of these things appeal to you then planting a tree or plant of some sort often pleases him.

So you need a sterile blade or needle if you plan on doing this.

Cernunnos doesn't seem to have any Vampire-like qualities so I

Hunting

would deem it less dangerous to offer him a part of your life force.

You will need a censer and some incense. If you can gather some dry moss or dry leaves etc to burn on it from the place you are using, all the better. Any woody or musty aromas seem to please him.

You don't have to dress in any particular manner but I think it best to use natural fibres rather than man made.

Fire and water are not essential and it is probably safer to avoid anything inflammable in forests especially in the summer months but it is up to you. If you prefer all four basic elementals to be represented then by all means go for it, safely.

Choose a quiet place where you are pretty sure you won't be disturbed and leave the place as you found it. This shows more respect in public places. If you plan to use your own land or garden it is a different matter and you can go to any lengths you wish to honour Cernunnos.

It seems that Cernunnos, like Ing and The Green Man came from the East and travelled west. So you might want to face east if wishing to draw something to you through him or west if asking for help to banish something.

Hold your symbolic hunting weapon whilst calling him. Choose any stance you feel is right on the day, e.g. standing, sitting etc.

Open yourself up energetically and spend a few minutes imagining him and when you feel ready call.

The Calling

I call upon Cernunnos Lord of the hunt, King of the forest creatures, he who has dominion over our wilder forces.

Hear me, as I sit here in your space and wait patiently for your arrival, hear my heart beating, hear my breath as it goes gently in and out, feel my energy as it pulls you to me.

Cernunnos whose being is at one with the forest landscape and the beasts that live within, Cernunnos whose life force permeates to us the human children for whom he has made his presence felt.

Accept this incense as I burn it in your honour to cleanse this space from any unwanted spirits or harmful forces

Hail Cernunnos, he who strides through the trees as a giant above those whom he hunts and whose cloven hooves leave no mark upon the ground.

Hail, Cernunnos, the peaceful one whose presence tames all the wild beasts and stills the air around him.

Hail Cernunnos, the fertile, the symbol of male sexuality, the force of nature made man for our souls to blend with.

Hail Cernunnos, whose antlers touch the tops of trees and whose eyes see all and whose ears hear all and whose strength and muscular form is like no other man or beast, dead or alive.

Hail Cernunnos, who aids the great hunt, whose presence means we are either the hunters or the hunted, help us to catch and avoid capture.

Hail Cernunnos, God of the free, the liberated, the rich beyond measure, the healthy and strong, the wildness of the deep forest and the keeper of the hidden secrets that lie beyond the mist and veils.

Here my/our call and come to me/us this…….(fill in as required e.g. this winters morn) accept this our offering to you and know that if we give you our blood it is in the hope you will aid us in our hunt.

Give your offering and sit patiently in meditation and await signs of his presence. If you are giving of your blood let a few drops fall onto the ground or roots of a tree.

Once you feel he is with you it is time to give your thanks and ask for anything you wish him to do for you.

Once you feel the communion has finished, close by thanking him for all he has shared and bid him farewell.

To add further energy to this ritual you can make love if in a couple and think of something you both wish for at the moment of climax.

If not wishing to give him your sexual energy you can support local or global green issues, especially forest related, or plant a tree in his honour. All of this will add to your magic.

CHAPTER THREE
Tattooing and Associated Practices

Tattooing and cutting the skin during ritual or for religious or spiritual purposes is an intense matter. It is a very ancient practice and taking it a step further and leaving dye impregnated most probably stems from initiation rites where people would be cut and herbs or ochre and other such materials were pressed into the wound. The blood aspect ties the person to the deity they have bled for.

The earliest concrete evidence for deliberate permanent incised pigmentation of human skin can be found from as far back as 30,000 BCE. However early Neanderthals left evidence of tool making, jewellery and perforated body art and they were most probably doing this as way back as 120,000BCE. The first images found in places such as Polynesia seem to be achieved by utilising charcoal and sharp bones. With cave art dating back as far as 50,000 years BCE we know mankind became artistic very early on in his development. Most of the earliest art depicts hunting scenes and we know from continued tribal practises that primitive man also adorned his skin with paint before going off to hunt or to war. These temporary markings had their purposes. One acted as camouflage and is still used to this day by armed forces and the other worked to intimidate the enemy. But why go from this easy to wash off tradition to actually incising the skin and laying down permanent pigment? This isn't immediately clear. It did, however, catch on more in some cultures than others. Some suggest it was due to increased inter tribal friction and skirmishes that led to each tribe wanting distinctive identification over neighbouring rivals. This might be partly why so many varied forms of scarification, tattooing, implants and piercings evolved. Even today we can see evidence for this in African tribes and other traditional tribal customs all over the world. This individual tribal symbolism caught on and to this day is still a big part of why people have tattoos. They become identified by them.

The pain people are prepared to go through seems to be a rite of passage, and we see this echoed right up until present day. Many a young person cannot wait to get their first piercing or tattoo, it is very popular. It has also been suggested that tattooing has its roots in shamanic practises and this could also be very true. What ever the reasons whether they are simply artistic, for hunting, war, rites of passage or shamanic, it appears that mankind has had a very long history of cutting and bleeding deliberately, making us unique in the animal kingdom as a whole. And those who think there isn't much blood in this obviously haven't watched one being done or had one themselves, it is bloody business. People having tattoos describe it as either getting new 'ink' or being 'cut' and that is exactly what it is. One thing I have noticed is the growth in popularity among the pagan and occult community where tattooing is concerned. The middle and upper class snobbery connected to it seems to be diminishing and now people from all walks of life are getting inked.

When the 'Ice Mummy' was found perfectly preserved high in the Oetz valley in Austria his 5,200 year old body amazed people who were fascinated by the tattooed dots all over this body. They tallied with acupuncture points and appeared to be almost like a permanent prescription. This incredible find hadn't been seen before but it doesn't mean that he is the only example of it merely that he is the only example that has so far been discovered. We already know that acupuncture goes back many thousands of years and as our earliest form of meridian therapy it is still being investigated by scientists today, all keen to try and explain its effectiveness. But it is accepted in mainstream Western medicine these days because put simply, it works.

Tattooing and other forms of permanent skin incision art represent a commitment, whether it is to your tribe, spiritual beliefs and/or healing requirements — it is taking a step beyond the temporary marking into a dedicated state of being. There are numerous spiritual and family traditions connected with tattooing. From taking on the family 'marks' before marriage, as in the customs of Hainan where a woman must be tattooed just before her wedding with her new husbands marks clearly imprinted upon her face, to Fijians who believe un-tattooed women minus pierced ears are to be struck down by the deceased souls of other women and offered up to the Gods as a sacrifice.

The aboriginal tattooing traditions are rife and mostly seem to be methods that people found, or still to this day find, to sign their blood allegiance with their tribe, families and belief systems. These blood rites are some of the oldest we have left of much earlier traditions and are still practiced today. These beliefs go further than skin deep. Many people have them done to appease deities and ancestors and to enable the deceased soul to be recognised in the afterlife, as many believe they retain a recognisable form comparable to their living body after death. Hindus believe this — they are extremely superstitious about tattoo marks surviving death. This is also a way of identifying a caste. Many have temporary henna tattoos but permanent ones are just as prevalent.

There is a strong global belief that whilst you undergo your tattoo and literally bleed for your family, deity etc. your energy, and the tattoo, is transmitted into the spirit world. The tattoo is not only imprinted into your skin it also makes its mark on inner planes of existence. To mark yourself with ink in this way is to mark your soul for eternity. A person may undergo a ritual in order to discover their animal totem and then decide to have a tattoo of it on their skin to further strengthen the bond. This practise is another common source of applied protection and/or magical healing. It makes direct contact with the spirit of the totem and links that individual with it forever. North American Indians are famous for this and frequently believe the tattoo is a way of always having the power of the animal and/or spirit represented in the image and that it is impossible to remove from the person. This is another clue as to why tattooing is so popular among many early cultures.

Our early hunter gatherer ancestors travelled light. Extraneous objects were a burden and jewellery can be lost, broken or stolen so a permanent mark on a person's skin is one thing that enables them to carry power and influence without any effort whatsoever. If you believe in the power of such protection, it is an incredible way of creating psychological and magical security at all times. But rites of passage are equally marked in this way. From a girl starting her periods to a boy dropping his testicles, to the birth of a baby, or a warrior about to fight in his first battle; all have a history of tattooing associated with them. There hardly seems to be a single rite of passage that doesn't have a history of tattooing linked to it and here in the UK we are no exception. Some of our Celtic tribal ancestors covered themselves in woad before battle. This blue dye madespeople appear as if they were the walking dead and terrified the enemy. The dye was also mixed with other ingredients which when applied to the skin give it an almost antiseptic quality. One can see distinct advantages here. Not only were you able to freak out your enemy by being naked and blue but your wounds healed better in many cases.

Wounds are another explanation for deliberate scarification. When we gain a cut or abrasion it sometimes it leaves a mark, and this mark is a constant reminder of the event. Each time we look at it we are taken back to the moment we gained it. These non-deliberate invasions might also have had accompanied infections and fevers through which if the person survived he might have experienced delirium. This delirium is similar to the altered states sought by the shaman. And visions can occur in these moments, flash backs and ancestral associations occur. These would have had a profound effect on the ancient primitive brain. The resulting scar had a story attached to it. And around the fire our ancestors would tell tales of their war wounds, much as people still do to this day — it seems almost instinctive behaviour. But why people went from historical enactments to deliberate marks made in cold blood with no particular tale associated is not clear and, as we have seen, may have many roots and reasons.

In some respects the global tradition of 'blood brothers' fallsunder this banner. Although it is by and large a male preserve it probably has very old roots. Young men often seem drawn to do this in their teens. This blood brother bond is taken seriously and in some respects one imagines its roots were in bands of hunters and warriors. The blood pact is meant to link the people concerned for life in an unbreakable loyal bond. They each cut themselves, usually on the palm or arm, and then press their wounds together allowing the blood to mix. This blending of each others blood and the swearing of an oath of allegiance is taken very seriously. Great loyalty is from thence on expected from each blood brother. And this is continued for life. The Romans, Scythians, and Norse men all had versions of it. A famous one took place in Norman times.

Robert d'Ouilly and Roger d'Ivry were two Norman knights who descended upon our shores during the Norman conquest of 1066. They were well known as blood brothers. Having both survived Hastings they were granted lands in Oxfordshire. As they had agreed prior to the invasion to split any proceeds they gained if they survived the battle, the lands were shared. Wallingford Castle was one project the blood brothers built together. The scar that such a bond creates is a reminder of the loyalty to each other, for as long as it lasts.

Many mummies discovered in Egypt are tattooed in one way or another. Most seem of spiritual significance. They often resemble marks associated with the deity of the family concerned. Tattoos relating to the Goddess Hathor, for example, are frequently imitations of pregnancy stretch marks. In fact the vast majority of tattooed mummies from Egypt seem to be female and have fertility and/or sexual connotations.

Egyptian men also had deliberate body modifications, the most popular and longest lasting of all of them being the practise of circumcision. It is believed that this began in Egypt and was adopted by the Hebrews through Abraham and his covenant with God. Its original purpose seems partially lost in the mists of time, though evidence suggests it was an act associated with the spiritual elite of the time, the priesthood. Considering Egyptian priests removed all body hair and were expected to enter the temples clean and pure of body, it isn't a monumental leap of imagination to see them one day deciding on a new exclusive rite of passage. It is well known that many a young man did a period of initiation into priesthood and this could be equated with a sort of religious national service much akin what to the practice of building great pyramids and monuments became during the dry season. If you wanted a more permanent method of marking this rite, what better than some form of body mutilation? It caught on and soon became the norm for both the priesthood and the male elite. Abraham was alleged to have been 93 when he was circumcised but he knew the significance and the effect it would have on his tribe. And though today it is often carried out for hygiene and medical reasons, it is still a tradition among the Jewish peoples and is very popular in America where most men are circumcised.

Ask anyone today why they are having tattoos and they will have a reason. Even if that reason is purely because they were drunk and dared by a friend it is a reason. Bravery seems to have much to do with it. Anyone who has been tattooed will tell you, it hurts. The needle pierces the skin deeply enough to make it bleed and stain the underlying layers with ink. If you watch someone having a tattoo it is surprising to see how much they bleed. And though modern inks are far more sophisticated than urine and soot, a favoured method utilised by South American tribes, it still carries a risk.

There are different types of tattooists. Some are called 'scratchers' these amateur tattooists haven't completed an apprenticeship or qualified. Some are decidedly dodgy and lack proper hygiene facilities or precautions and are best avoided at all costs. Most people will advise you to always go to a recognised professional parlour but some scratchers are safe. Many a 'scratcher' takes proper hygiene precautions, but you are taking a big risk and I certainly wouldn't pay a 'scratcher' to practice on my skin. But I have allowed an apprentice tattooist to give me two tattoos.

It is not generally known that the modern day tattoo gun owes its birth to a hole punching device originally designed to make holes in paper. Thomas Edison created that device and Samuel O'Reilly patented his tattoo gun in 1891 having been inspired by Edisons puncher. The repetitive action allows the needle to be inserted in and out of the skin at such speed that as the tattooist drags the gun across the skin it perforates and cuts. The ink is fed down through the needle but the action of the gun allows it to literally create a pump action that facilitates the incision and insertion of the ink. Each colour change requires a change of needle and/or sterilising in between. Most tattooists will begin with darker colours first and end with the lighter ones. If they go too deep you might experience scarring and possible ink-leakage, or 'bleeding' into surrounding skin. This is partly where experience will always have the advantage. If they don't go deep enough then the ink might not take and you will have to go back for touch up sessions. Each person's skin is slightly different but an experienced tattooist will recognise your type and make allowances for it. Younger skin varies from older skin; people who work outdoors often develop leathery skin and very old people often have thin skin. These factors all need considering.

Piercing is also more popular than ever before. For many years in modern society we became familiar with women getting their ears pierced and for a long time this remained the most popular and fashionable Western tradition. But now it is another explosive trend for men and women alike. And no part of the body is being ignored in this practise. From labia and penises to weaved and threaded spines to facial and tongue piercings they are everywhere. It is another market where hygiene must be paramount and professionalism imperative if you wish to minimalize risks associated with it but that said, many a piercing happens spontaneously. And it is another tradition with very primitive roots. It seems that subconsciously many of us today are being drawn back to the primal and tribal.

Some of the most extreme examples can be seen in tribes who pierce the lips of their women and then expect them to gradually increase the hole gained by placing larger and larger clay plates in them. These women look grotesque by our standards as they go about their business wearing these often huge objects hanging by stretched lower lips. While flesh rings on ears are gaining more popularity in our Western culture, I can't see lip plates catching on.

Piercing has been used for many reasons over our mutual human history. It was often used by South American tribes, among others, as a form of punishment. By inflicting great pain on the perpetrator you re-gained submission to the laws of the society and made sure the community knew there were negative consequences for misconduct. Mayan priests often self-mutilated as a way of showing subservience to their Gods and offering their blood.

There seem to be many reasons for people to have tattoos and piercings. Here are a few we've touched upon:

Cultural tradition
Magical protection
Religious significance
Rite of passage
Tribal identification
Family identification
Afterlife beliefs
Healing
Sexual/fetish
Purely aesthetic
Peer pressure
Fertility

With this number of reasons, some of which are extremely ancient and deeply entrenched in our psyches, it is no wonder that both tattooing and piercings have continued to flourish.

Having a protection tattoo is one that crosses pretty much all cultural divides and is still one of the most popular acquired by people today. These sorts of markings vary considerably, from specific sigils to particular words to superstitious images or pictures often of animals, birds or fish; protection is big business and always has been. One part of the body that seems the most popular for locating protection tattoos is the back. By literally 'covering ones back' one can feel safer.

The south-east Asian practice of *Yantra* or *Sak Yant*, meaning 'to tap', is very popular. Carried out by Buddhist monks who are also well versed in magical abilities not too far removed from what many might describe as 'witchcraft', it is predominantly used for protection. The tattoos are mainly placed upon the back of the client. They don't use a tattoo gun but employ a far older method of utlising a long narrow bamboo stick that has a sharp point to it and dipping it in specially prepared magical ink. The symbols are meditated on before hand so the monk knows in advance what the client needs in the way of a tattoo. The client will be expected to visit the monk prior to getting his tattoo so tthat he monk can do this. This is now catching on with tourists, especially in places such as Cambodia and Singapore.

This sort of protection is very common — one takes an image associated with a protective influence in your life and utilises it in this way. It doesn't always matter if you can actually see your tattoo every day, simply knowing it is there and what it looks like and symbolises to you works the desired magic you seek. And it doesn't stop at the place or type of symbol or image; often tattooists would incorporate magical ingredients into their ink. The precise make up of most tattoo inks are a closely guarded secret. And to this day it is possible to find people using magical potions in their mixtures.

The Burmese have a long-standing history of using magical ingredients in ink, especially where love is concerned. They usually advise and encourage sexually active couples to have cabbalistic symbols and images in black and red on their bodies to increase the tantric connection between the couple. By enhancing their sex lives through magical permanent markings, the couple are creating stronger bonds and have much greater chances of maintaining a long lasting union. The ink for this particular practise is always potent with magical extras. The incredibly strong belief that this tradition works is probably most of the magic, but I for one would not undermine any of these traditions or belittle them, and personally do believe in many of their inherent mysterious claims.

Tattooing as a form of healing has a very long standing tradition in many cultures, from branding a baby, to curing a convulsion, to simply enduring extremely long, drawn out tattoos. Using the pain to cleanse and clear the effects of another pain is common and all kinds of tattoos and brandings are used. In some respects tattooing is just another form of bloodletting. A belief that illness and pain are all symptomatic of evil spirits and demons perpetuates among the vast majority of ancient pagan cultures and indigenous tribal customs. The idea of banishing the evil by causing more pain seems mad, but, as an idea, it often works. Quite often if we as human beings are in one sort of pain, having another entirely different pain inflicted deliberately in another part of the body often confuses the mind, distracts from the first pain and can give temporary relief. Many shamans would gain enough success here because if you then add the patient's trust and belief in the shaman's methods to cure him or her, you have another big psychological plus on the road to healing.

The most well known form of healing with needles, though not necessarily those that have ink, is acupuncture. This is slightly different however. And though the skin is pierced and can bleed during treatment no permanent mark will remain afterwards. But the incredible effects of stimulating these meridians on the body that connect through the nervous system with the basic flow of chi/energy throughout the person has several thousand years of successful application behind it.

The Maori people are synonymous with permanent body markings. These people have a very long standing spiritual and cultural tradition of tattooing, often from head to toe, but are most famous for their incredible facial art. Like many tribal peoples they incorporate traditional hunting images, fertility ones, and use red as a way of marking death or taboos. Women often stain their lips black once they are successful in having children as it marks them as fertile and adult. The Maori art often seeks balance and symmetry on the body so images are repeated equally on both sides. This is a practise found in most Australian and New Zealand areas. They also had a slave population for a while and would shave the head of the slave and tattoo him or her so that the owner would be instantly recognised. This practise extended to branding, another tradition that is gaining in modern popularity in a voluntary capacity. It is ironic, in some respects, that the very acts we once thought of as barbaric and demeaning are now sought after by individuals who do actually have a choice and freedoms. It was also common among these aboriginal peoples to lean towards complex geometric designs and spirals. The artist would be highly skilled and trained with the potential to gain a good standing in the community and always receive good remuneration. If the tattooist was unhappy with the client in any way or felt he would be unable to pay the appropriate fee then he could mark his feelings with badly drawn lines and smudged colours; a tattooist has your skin as his canvas and will mark you for life so it pays to treat him with respect and pay his fee without question.

Another group of people from all over the world who are well known for their love of tattoos are seamen. There are hardly any sailors past or present who haven't got at least one tattoo. Those who live their lives on the oceans waves encounter many differing countries and traditions along the way. This is most probably how people from countries with less of a tattooing background first discovered body art. The drunken sailor coming home from his first trip with his tattoo became something the nautical world took to like ducks to proverbial water, if you'll excuse the pun. Some common popular designs include clasped hands, anchors, a naked woman, a ship, etc. They have a strong tradition of showing their love for women through their tattoos. This isn't surprising considering they would often be away at sea for months on end their opportunities with the opposite sex were less than the land lovers. So whether their tattoo represented their love that is left behind on shore or a love they aspire to meeting on leave, images of women, particularly dancing ones, are very popular and common among them. Military men also have a fondness for gaining the tattoo of their regiment and/or commemorative markings to friends they have lost in action.

The bloodletting aspect of tattooing is minimal but the sensation of being cut intense. And the overwhelming feeling of connection with so many of your fellow human beings whilst having the ink injected is strong, primal and ancient. It is no wonder those who have one often have more.

I doubt if there are many Gods or Goddesses, Angels or demons, ancestors or fae, lwa or saints that have been missed out when it comes to people having permanent dedicated markings or marks associated with them. So to find a God of tattooing is nigh on impossible as you can have a tattoo to represent anything that an artist is capable of interpreting.

Some people seem to rush into getting tattoos and some give it careful consideration. If yours is to be of a spiritual or religious significance it is generally believed that the deity, entity, etc. will recognise it and sense its presence around you. You will also be taking this image to the grave with you and as you die, leaving your shell behind, the imprint of your tattoo or scar will be acknowledged across the veil. So with this in mind, for those who believe in this, it will pay to give it very serious consideration. You are showing your allegiance and this is forever.

I see the actual tattoo or scarification being the ritual, and naturally it can also be part of a bigger ritual or initiation or rite of passage, so I don't feel there is any real need to perform a separate one unless you feel you should of course.

We can learn from the Buddhist monks here. It does help to have a pre-tattoo mediation, if you are the sort of person to practice meditating. And also drawing a rough impression of the planned image and sleeping with it under your pillow might help you gain a greater subconscious connection with it.

But other than this I feel it better to avoid giving any particular examples of rituals here.

Tattoo Meditation

I deem this safe for most people to replicate if they wish to but it is probably best to avoid it if you are asthmatic, have lung disease or allergies to incense.

Before taking that massive step towards your first tattoo it might pay off to do this meditation. And if needing inspiration for a tattoo, this is also of use.

Choose a quiet undisturbed time and allow about 15-30 minutes.

Have a bath or shower to rid yourself of the energies you've accumulated prior to the meditation.

Get comfortable, preferably sitting or in the lotus position.

Light some white candles and some heady incense — the sort that aids trance.

Take a few deep breaths and relax.

Now focus on your solar plexus and stay aware of it as you breathe slowly in and out. Take long and slow breaths for a few minutes.

Keep your focus on your solar plexus and after a few minutes stagger your inward breath, so breathe in for the count of four and out to the count of two. If this is difficult try 6/4.

After a few minutes of doing this, begin to allow your torso to gently sway either left to right or backwards and forwards or circular. This needs to be a slight sway.

Restore your breathing to normal but keep swaying and then either imagine the design you have planned, and see if anything more connected with it comes up in your mind's eye, or ask to be shown what you should get.

If you have problems with maintaining the breathing rhythm don't worry too much. This is just an easy way to get into a mild trance like state which is all you wish to achieve.

Don't force the breathing pattern. If it isn't easy to do then just keep the breathing gentle and shallow once you begin swaying.

Once you've seen enough, stop swaying.

Take a long deep breath afterwards before standing up.

You might find you need to eat and drink something to ground yourself after.

CHAPTER 4
Vampires

Vampires, creatures of the night, nocturnal blood drinking undead beings that haunt the earth. Do they exist, and if so in what form?

We've all heard of Vampires and possibly watched many a film and maybe read many a book on the subject. One thing most people will agree upon, there is something incredibly fascinating with these nocturnal bloodsuckers. But where did Vampires originate from and is it really some old Transylvanian Count Dracula whose tragic love story began the myth? Well probably not as he was most likely to have been inspired by the infamous Count Vladimir otherwise known as 'Vlad the Impaler'.

He was born as Prince Vladimir of Wallachia in 1431, of Hungarian nobility. His father was a member of the Order of the Dragon and his name was Dracula, meaning 'the son of the dragon'. This became his name also. During his family's campaigns against the Ottoman Empire, he was known for the delight he took in torturing his victims, and his pride in high death tolls. Having been abused and beaten regularly by his military trainers, he developed a taste for pain — preferably other people's suffering. He is best known for impaling his captors on large wooden spikes causing a long, drawn out and excruciatingly painful death. This blood thirsty man with the Dracula name was adopted by Bram Stoker who was inspired by his life. The family were descended from Transylvanian Saxons which provided him with a location for the story. Apart from his warring, Vlad wasn't a bloodsucker. Nor did he rise up after death.

There have always been ancient stories of demons, spirits and 'undead' rising up and seeking to feed on the living. These myths persist throughout nearly every culture but none captured the imaginations of the general populous quite like the blood sucking Vampire. And as the stories of these creatures spread from the Balkans and other parts of Eastern Europe over the last few hundred years, so writers caught them in their literary nets and weaved their words into the popular novels we are familiar with today.

The first to write on Vampires were the Babylonians with their terrifying *labartu* — a female demon who had a particular taste for the blood of children, though she would quite happily feast on adults and animals also. She most likely evolved from the Sumerian Goddess Lamashtu who had the same attributes and was also known as Lambartu. The Hebrew Lilith also gets called Queen of the Vampires by modern neo-pagans. She is often seen as a succubus and baby killer. My own opinion is that the modern Queen of Vampires is a composite of several other beings or entities including the Assyrian storm demon Lilitu, the Akkadian succubus Ardat-lili and the baby killing Sumerian Lamashtu. So it wasn't such a leap of imagination to then cast her as a Vampire ,and there she has remained in the popular psyche of today. These stories also seemed to spread into the Greek and Roman psyche with their own *lamiae,* who preyed more specifically on young men. Each Vampire seems to have its preference. Not all Vampires are exclusively blood drinkers, some

Vampires

like to eat the flesh of their victims! Others are the seemingly more socially acceptable 'energy Vampires'. The varying types of Vampires that have arisen over time all have one thing in common: they all seem to stem from unaccountable deaths and the fear invoked by the required explanation of these happenings.

The Romanians have a word to describe Vampires and it is *strigoi*. These were thought to rise up from their homes on the steep sided Carpathian mountains and fly by night to their unsuspecting victims. Anyone who has visited this area will tell you it has retained its medieval architecture and does boast some impressive castles clinging to its cliffs but the locals will groan at the mention of Dracula. Some Tourism does exist to perpetuate the myth and cash in on the tale but it is just that, a tale, and probably nothing more.

In eighteenth century Europe it was common to blame certain unexplainable events on Vampires. It became almost commonplace to have exhumations of corpses to make sure they really were dead. Ghosts took on a more sinister dark and twisted side by suddenly developing a taste for human blood and would drain it from their victims whilst they slept. All sorts of superstitions arose from these hysterical beliefs. Fear of the 'undead' spread like wildfire across Eastern Europe and from stillborn babies to suicides all had the capacity to be Vampires.

The pale complexion often taken on by people with anaemic conditions wasn't explainable to people without medical knowledge or modern scientific understanding. People made assumptions on diagnosis. If someone who was previously healthy gradually became lethargic and eventually exhausted for no obvious reason then Vampirism gave them an explanation. Modern day anaemia is now explained and we have cures for it but back in the days when malnutrition was commonplace and mortality rates much higher, where modern science hadn't yet evolved, people turned to their priests. The priests needed to give their people reasons for the terrible things occurring. So they looked to witches, dead or alive, and anyone who might seem a little odd or out of the ordinary in life. They had to come up with something and so anything that was potentially evil, dark or the Devil's work would do nicely.

Many superstitious practices evolved around Vampires with each country having its own variations. In Eastern Europe throughout the renaissance to the early nineteenth century there was a major focus on Vampire activity. It became popular to place bodies upside down in coffins to prevent them from becoming Vampires and leaving their resting places. The etymology of the word Vampire seems to have stemmed from the Russian *Upir Lyklyi* meaning, 'wicked Vampire'. The Russians were particularly keen on pointing the finger towards those they believed were former witches in life as being the reason for Vampirism in their society. But it wasn't until John Polidon wrote his novel The Vampyre in 1819 that we meet the first truly explored fictional character of the Vampire that has become more commonplace today. At a much later date Bram Stoker's novel Dracula in 1897 sealed the modern Vampire's fate, becoming the benchmark for all vampire stories of today.

Here we meet the concepts of Vampires creating new Vampires, their need to stay out of the light, sleeping in coffins by day and all the other characteristics of the Vampire that we all know. As well as drawing from the life of Vlad the Impaler, Bram Stoker probably took some of his inspiration from his own backyard in Ireland. The Dearg-due, who is also known as Dearg-dul, Dearg- dililat and Dearg-diylai, was a young woman forced into an arranged marriage. As if it wasn't bad enough that she had to relinquish her own chosen love, she ended up being badly abused by her husband. Eventually, so the story goes, she committed suicide. Not long after this people began reporting that they'd seen her. Some saw her at the anniversary of her death each year, some several times a year, and some say she roams at each full moon. She seems to have all the qualities we associate with succubae merged with the undead appearance of the Vampire. She is accused of preying on young men whilst they sleep, seducing them and draining them of their 'life force'. Now whether this refers to blood or semen isn't clear in any sources I've found but it is more likely to be blood as the term 'life force' usually pertains to this.

Another name synonymous with the Vampire legend is Erzebeth Bathory. Born in 1560 of Hungarian descent, her brother was Voivod of Transylvania. Her official title was Countess Erzebeth Bathory de Ecsed and after she married Ferenc Nadasdy she went to live in Castle Nadasdy in Sarvor. Her husband died and she was left alone to rattle around the castle with few for company. But the few she did have were to become her allies. It is said that they became torturers and murderers of young women in one of the most infamous serial killing sprees there have ever been. She and her cohorts were accused of killing hundreds of local girls. This does not always tally up with her outward behaviour. Yes she was rich and powerful but she also championed women's rights. She was eventually caught out and convicted of killing 80 and then sent to live in solitary confinement for the rest of her life. The only reason it is thought that she escaped the death sentence was because of her status and the need to avoid an even bigger scandal. It has been suggested that her interfering nature and her habit of sticking up for women gave her enemies ammunition they used for their own devices, and that they then turned her love of her own sex into something more grotesque and macabre.

The stories that abounded after her death were incredible. There were tales of her bathing in the blood of the young victims and actually drinking the blood in a deluded belief that she might gain immortality and eternal youth. None of these were ever proven nor were they the actual crimes she was accused of. So was she a blood-drinking Vampire who loved to torture her essentially female victims or was she a feminist? We might never know the entire truth of what happened in the castle but she was known to have been a good wife and mother but with a lesbian lust. Stories of wild lesbian orgies, also involving her aunt, abounded and at some point she took her erotic desires to their extreme. When I think of the average dominatrix today with her dungeon and instruments of playful torture, Erzebeth Bathory comes to mind. Maybe she delighted in exploring her erotic nature and found others that also shared her lusts?

It was said by her accusers that her bloodlust began just after she killed for the first time and noticed that where the blood of her virgin victim had splattered onto her skin it appeared younger and firmer afterwards. This is what provoked, if we are to believe it, her extreme motivation for blood. She is alleged to have constructed all manner of torturous machines including an iron maiden with internal spikes to gain the enormous amounts of blood she required. But again this was hearsay and could be a gross exaggeration of what was really a harmless sexual dungeon device. Her accomplices were executed and she was imprisoned in Slovakia and died there. After her death they found many uneaten meals and empty glasses, leading her captors to think she was starved of blood and died because of it. In truth she was probably just old and frail and died of natural causes. But her unique and bizarre history captures the imaginations of many and it is entirely possible that her life was partly responsible for the Carpathian Castle and blood bath connections of the later Vampire books that emerged in the nineteenth centuries. Whatever her motivation or actual actions she has left us with a rich tapestry to weave our blood tales with.

But we have to ask, are there really blood sucking people out there? And if so, why do they do it? The answer to this is, yes there are and the answer to why each of them participates in this act may vary. There seem to be three types of modern day Vampire.

Vampires

One is the psychic Vampire, who will probe your mind and plant information that they hope you will act upon. They are able to draw images and energy from your third eye if it is not closed or protected. This can vary from something as innocuous as the dieting Vampire wishing to have her cake and eat it, by being able to share your enjoyment of said food through psychic invasion, to the more deliberately evil and manipulative variety. But this sort of Vampire is hard to prove and therefore if they do exist, and I for one believe that they do, they can hide behind convention very easily and make anyone accusing them seem paranoid. The easiest thing to do with this sort of unwanted behaviour is to avoid the person like the plague or put up enough psychic defence as to render them impotent in your life. It is interesting to note that when you protect yourself adequately they often lose interest in you as you no longer provide them with a food source.

The second form of Vampire is the naive energy Vampire. This person is similar to the psychic one but might not be aware of their true nature. They need other people's energy to function at their optimum. These people are often the sort that will leave you feeling drained if you spend time with them. It is as though the energy pendulum takes a swing whilst you are there. This sort of Vampire normally needs to be in actual physical company of its potential 'food bag' to feed. As their energy lifts so yours will fall and an effective Vampire can drain you in under an hour should they wish. And this will happen every time you have anything to do with them. They literally suck the life force from you. They may be aware of their nature and if so it won't make any difference because their urge to feed will override their conscience. Some people are happy to be a 'food bag' for such folk but this is rare. I advise taking the same precautions and actions as with the psychic Vampire.

The last variety is more true to type in that this is the Vampire who craves blood. Some will claim an uncontrollable desire for blood that has always been there. Blood, like any substance you may or may not taste, is an acquired taste. Some people faint at the mere sight of it but some are attracted to it. Basically, some people like the taste of blood. There is a long history of drinking blood and there are many tribes in Africa that still partake of it. These are people drinking the blood of their cattle from time to time to supplement their diet. The cattle are put into trance and their throat is cut just enough to allow blood to drain. They only take that which they need and don't normally kill the animal this way unless it is meant to be sacrificed for food. The regular bloodletting normally leaves the animal perfectly healthy afterwards. Too much blood in the stomach will make you wretch so it is only meant as an iron rich supplement. This sort of blood drinking is nothing whatsoever to do with Vampires but goes to show that as a practice it still occurs in some cultures to this day.

An exceptional variety of modern Vampires are Strigoi VII. This 'Family' of Vampires claim a sanguine heritage. Though Vampires in many ways, they do not take or drink each others blood. For them, blood is a metaphor for energy, yet if you were to accuse them of being merely energy Vampires they would be offended and deny it. This family seem more subtle and esoteric in nature. They do have many of the traditions associated with Vampires, including the donning of artificial canines and a certain style of dress that one might see as gothic or fetish inspired, but they are not openly declaring a literal taste for the red stuff. As a mystery tradition, they have drawn on many varied influences from the occult world, literature and myths and legends. They are encouraged to seek self-mastery, which they feel will lead to greater enjoyment and appreciation of life, and definitely advocate treating the body as a temple of ultimate pleasure. Many things one associates with modern life are not seen as beneficial to a happy life and these are fast foods, computer games, TV, or addictions of any sort. But literature, the arts, music and good food are all encouraged and one can understand why. The theory being that the aim is to balance and find equilibrium and harmony in all things in life betwixt day, night and twilight 'times'. These they see as representing the conscious material day life, and the subconscious spiritual ethereal night life and the turning point of twilight or liminal life, with each time having its inherent mysteries or secrets to reveal to ones self and how one wants to master each aspect. There is also much talk of immortality and the key to it being a holy grail to aspire to. This is indeed a mystery school with firm foundations should one wish to join it and partake of the inner secrets, but as with any magical training, it is not without risks and sometimes the journeys we take within are the most difficult to achieve with any degree of success. And sometimes opening up greater awareness can lead to madness should the person be pre-disposed to instability or neurosis. It also seems to indicate that only certain people have the 'blood' this being the main mention of it indicating a particular inherent tendency towards being part of this particular 'family'. One feels one waits to be approached rather than approaching them, and in some ways this retains the older closed circle nature of the revival mystery school traditions.

The modern day blood-taking Vampire is after one thing only, your blood. And in these times of AIDS and Hepatitis among other blood born diseases it is easy to see that the practise is fraught with danger. There are clubs and closed groups that do indulge in this activity but again they are very rare. There are a plethora of web sites dedicated to the practise and some give sensible advice on sanguine activities while others are ill informed. Menstrual blood is also categorised here as even oral sex can spread diseases and strengthen blood ties. Be warned. This might seem abhorrent and disgusting but, as I mentioned in chapter one, menstrual blood has a very long magical history. There are many myths concerning types of blood and what the signs and symptoms of vampirism are. Let us look at each one individually.

All Vampires are nocturnal — Some lean towards this but often have to fight against it because of the need to fit into society. There is no hard and fast rule here although you do find a lot of modern Vampires evolving from the Gothic world and they do seem to prefer night time.

All Vampires suck blood — Not true, actually very few do, at least on a regular basis. As mentioned there are many kinds of Vampire.

All Vampires have to sleep in coffins — Twaddle, they can if they wish to but each to their own.

All Vampires hate garlic, are frightened and disempowered by Holy water and run at the mere sight of a wooden stake, oh and wear inverted crucifixes and won't go into Churches — Again this is not true.

All Vampires have to wear black — Rubbish.

All Vampires have fangs — This does seem to be pre-requisite although not essential.

All Vampires have claws — Long nails do seem a part of the overall package, yes, but again, optional.

All Vampires are Satanists — Some are, some not. Some are Christian! Each Vampire has their own spiritual beliefs. In fact, the vast majority do seem to have had a Catholic upbringing.

All vampires are walking dead — I've yet to meet one.

Vampires have to have blood daily — Not true.

The most effective Vampires often blend so well into the background of life as to almost become invisible. This ability to me is true vampirism. Where the drinking of blood is concerned there is no absolute way you can assure yourself that the person you are taking blood from hasn't got a disease you could catch. You take just as much risk with this kind of behaviour as you do with having unprotected sex. Any forced bloodletting is a criminal offence and will potentially land you in jail; it will also serve to alienate you from others of your kind. If you must do it then at least use sterile lances and or needles. Options for these include sterilised blades of all sorts if sharp enough, diabetic needles, hypodermic needles. All should be disposable if possible and a sharps box is the best place for them. Avoid arteries for obvious reasons, if using a vein sterilise the skin first and only take very small amounts. You really don't need much to quell the craving, so I have been informed.

If it is a woman's menstrual blood you lust after then either get her to use a 'mooncup' to catch it in or drink directly, should she want you to of course. If including this in a consenting sexual practise it can be highly erotic. There is also a myth that drinking the combination of menstrual blood and semen is some sort of magical elixir and gateway to eternal youth. Elixir Rubeus is its official name. If involving it in a ritual sense, it can improve the effects of said magic dramatically. Sometimes all that is required is a scratch or small cut that a good taste can be gained from. You don't need to plunge too far into skin to make it bleed. There is another myth that a virgin's blood is the best, well it might well be — I could not say — but only from a virgin who is at least over 18.

Some cravings lead to animal blood and this is possible, not particularly nice but achievable. But don't go thinking your raw steak is full of blood, it isn't. The blood-like liquid in meat is not blood. It is a derivative of blood called myoglobin and is not going to give you the actual red blood cells you crave. So if a raw piece of meat is enough to calm your cravings, chances are, you are not a Vampire.

The mythical form of Vampire is a different beastie altogether. Once dead, it is given fresh un-life by another Vampire through bloodletting. The Vampire emerges after sundown to seek his or her prey. It is interesting to note that Vampires rarely seem to have preyed on the fit and healthy, preferring, it seems, to take from the weak and vulnerable. The Vampire is also seen as a shapeshifter able to fly with the wings of a bat, another nocturnal creature, in through open windows to its victims. It is meant to be very difficult to kill. Only a wooden stake through the heart or decapitation will end the Vampire's life, allegedly. All these elements conspire to create the more modern interpretation of the Vampire that we have today, and yet for all the Vampire's undead status and presumably rotten smell, it retains one characteristic that few other demons, Lilith apart, have. The Vampire is sexy. There is no getting away from it and I'm sure writers such as Anne Rice would agree having written so many Vampire stories. To those of a more dominant persuasion imagining yourself as the one who takes to the wing to land on the window ledge of your latest fancy and literally taking the life source from their neck, a very erogenous part of the body, is highly arousing. As is the counterpart submissive fantasy of waiting nervously not knowing if this quite often handsome stranger will arrive by night through your window to feast on your resting body makes for potent stuff — something writers, TV producers and Hollywood have all cashed in on. Vampires are big business.

Many of the roots that Vampires have evolved from have been determined by our obsession over death and the changing from one season to another. Death may be a taboo subject but it has more fascination to us than almost anything else we experience in life because of its absolute inevitability and the mysteries that surround it. And in an effort to link our own passing with the apparent death of life each Autumn means that it is no coincidence that the traditional 'Day of the Dead' is held at the beginning of November. The Celts have Samhain, and Christians All Souls or Saints day. This inevitable death of nature as winter takes hold is reflected in our own awareness of the transient nature of life. Each Halloween we remember our dead, dressing as the dead or as witches and creatures associated with the Moon and the night. Although in these technological times we have, for the most part, reduced our celebrations to trick-or-treat and maybe a party, the underlying awareness that this time of year throws our own mortality up into our faces is global. Ageing is inevitable, and yet vampires don't age. They have transcended death and become immortal for, as long as they can drink the blood of living creatures, their existence is guaranteed. The mere thought that there are people able to get up out of their graves and walk the earth at night has filled many a generation with fear and terror.

But what about ordinary everyday modern Vampires, surely they don't really drink each others blood? Yes they do. And whether it is between two consenting adults who, we hope, are aware of all the associated health risks or at a club especially for such people, they are doing it.

It wasn't difficult to choose a ritual for this chapter. I have been a child of Lilith all my life and probably past lives also. It seems an eternal link. She is definitely nocturnal and loves liminal spaces. One of her totems is the screech owl so she is on the wing at night. The mythology connecting her with Ardat Lili, the first recorded succubus of ancient Mesopotamia, is verified by many scholars. And she certainly loves her blood, so for your information only here is an example magical ritual to invoke Lilith.

Ritual to invoke and initiate into the Queen of Vampires — Lilith

This short ritual is for information only.

Lilith is primal and sexual and as such, blood and sex often come into a calling to her.

To prepare your altar, face it either east or south. Lilith comes from the Middle East in relation to the Western world and hers is the south wind so both of these directions will suffice. If you live in the southern hemisphere then face it towards the Middle East.

Place a red cotton or silk cloth upon it.

Prepare a fetish of Lilith in advance and dress her in red or give her red skin. Add wings to your fetish or use an image of her. Place this centrally.

Use six candles. Two black, two red and two white.

Make up an incense to honour her and offer up to her. This is one of the most powerful forces to draw Lilith to you. Use red sandalwood, with willow bark, spikenard, dried rose petals, and dry pomegranate seeds. This mix will give you a sound basic incense that she always seems to react to when burnt on a charcoal block.

Make sure artificial items are kept away from the altar and from yourself.

Pick deep red fragrant roses to offer her and if these are difficult to obtain then white lilies do just as well as she adores them.

Fill your chalice with red wine symbolic of the grail blood or use pure spring water consecrated with sea salt.

If it is possible place a skull, owl feathers and snake skin on the altar and a hand mirror face up but DO NOT LOOK INTO IT!!

Prepare yourself by taking a ritual bath and as with all my rituals use natural cloth, etc.

She appreciates items such as fresh pomegranates and figs and olives as food offerings.

Now you are ready.

The best times to call upon Lilith are at dusk and night time. Once the owls are out hunting, so is she.

The times when the moon is waxing gibbous and dark are best.

Open yourself up (raise your own witch energy) and as you do imagine Lilith in all her beautiful glory as a fiery red, voluptuous, loose haired Goddess, and be prepared to see her both as a creative and destructive force.

I call upon Lilith the south wind, the terrifying, the infertile and fertile, the baby killer and creator, the wife of God and Goddess of all you survey.

Mistress of the Vampires whose Star Fire burns like no other who can imbue her children with this element and allow them access to her secret realm

Come to me, your child, in this my hour of need.
Hail Lilith Predatory Queen of the night
Come to me in this my hour of need.
Hail Lilith lover and mistress of the stolen seed
Come to me in this my hour of need.
Hail Lilith, the succubus, and incubus
Come to me in this my hour of need.
Hail Lilith Queen of demons and divine inspiration
Come to me in this my hour of need.
Hail Lilith Sister of Lucifer the morning and evening star
Come to me in this my hour of need.
Hail Lilith consort of Samael
Come to me in this my hour of need.
Hail Lilith, keeper of the mirrors, seducer of Angels and Gods,
Come to me in this my hour of need.
Hail Lilith mother of Azaz-el the bound
Come to me in this my hour of need.
Feel my passions rise for you and Samael as I watch your infernal consummation

Protect me from the destructive force of your energy and invoke in me your love and lust.

Accept here my offerings of incense and wine and food in your honour and let me feel the eternal rhythm of your drum beat within my heart.

Cleanse me of impurities created by men and strengthen me against they who would choose to chain me. Let me be a free spirit on the southerly wind flying at your side in the darkness of the night.

Aid me in raising the serpent and allowing my energy to pull up from below as waves of your ecstatic bliss flow through me.

Oh Lilith most beautiful, most terrifying, most intelligent and most complex. You are a mother, a whore and harlot, you are, a primal force from before the beginning of time you are and the one men tremble most in the presence of, you are! She who finds her children through their life blood accept mine as I offer it unto you this night!

Now add more incense… continue drawing up the serpent kundalini energy not allowing it to spill over into the sexual (unless you are setting out to deliberately combine the energies of blood and sex, which is fine of course, then only give her that which you wish to).

Hail Lilith as you rise within me I am blessed by your continued inspiration, your gifts of creation, your demons, your Holy Spirit and filled with the wisdom of Sophia and in the Heaven of your angelic wings. Accept herein my eternal gratitude my libation to you of wine and food and mine own blood!

Make your blood offering onto the incense

Pour a few drops of wine over the fetish and symbolically offer her the food to eat.

Oh mother Lilith accept me, your child, as a new initiate keen to devote my time and life to your work, please let me pass across the void to you and find you in the darkness of mine own soul. Cradle me in your cold arms Lilith and know that it is my intention to honour and respect you and my wish to learn from you. Protect me from the destructive forces of your energy and allow me to bathe in ecstatic bliss as Samael , the serpent, winds his way into my fragile form. Help me to learn how best to use energy in all its forms. Feed me when there is no food to be had, love me when I am at my most alone, and heal me from the hurts of the past as I am born again in your Holy sight.

Now sit in quiet meditation and communion with her taking on board all images and sensations she bestows upon you. Never show any fear with Lilith regardless of what she does. If you have asked for her protection she is not going to do anything that would really hurt you but sometimes she likes to test initiates.

Once you feel the energy diminishing focus back on the altar and say.

Great and full of thanks in humbled devotion am I by your presence here tonight.

Enriched and blessed and released am I by your presence here tonight.

Loved and aroused and sated am I by your presence here tonight.

Honoured, loved and protected am I by your presence here tonight.

And now it is my wish to bid you my fondest and saddest farewell in this space tonight.

Farewell Lilith Queen of the Heavens and the night whose feathered wings can take flight once more in starry skies to fly freely where 'er it is her wish to be.

Farewell my Goddess and lover and mistress and greatest inspiration as you disappear once more over the horizon to seduce your lovers and feed on their seed.

Farewell Lilith the destroyer, the one between worlds, the liminal lady of the crossroads of life.

Farewell.

Now close down your chakras and let the candles burn themselves safely out. Eat the offerings and drink the wine in her honour and make notes of all you have experienced.

The two best moon phases for calling on Lilith are three days off full, when moon is waxing gibbous, and during the dark moon.

Offering Lilith both blood and sex regularly is not advised.

Keep the petals of the flowers on the altar to dry out and use in incenses in future as they will have her energy imbued within them.

Is best to bury the remnants of the incense.

CHAPTER 5
Human Sacrifices

Blood rituals and sacrifices can often mean different things. A blood ritual will involve blood but won't necessarily mean any life has been taken. Sacrifice however seems to imply both a greater reverence and that more has been given, usually a life. It is a ritual during which something we regard as sacred is let go of or offered up. For this reason I decided to have two separate chapters touching briefly on both subjects. This one is devoted to human sacrifice. Here we look at various cultural rituals involving the taking of a life in a religious or spiritual context. The next chapter looks at blood rituals of all sorts.

Our human history is steeped in these rituals. From the blood baths of the Aztecs to the roots of Christianity, ritual blood sacrifices have been made. Why our ancestors decided to make them isn't totally clear. The probable origins are due to our increased dependence on meat for food, and were a remnant of our Neolithic hunting rites.

Walter Burkett, a scholar on sacrifices, believes that blood sacrifices originated from the guilt of the kill. This could be a part of it. Our teeth have evolved to suit an omnivorous diet and we are most definitely both co-operative, peaceful creatures and barbaric, efficient killers. But I don't think it is as simple as guilt. Plenty of people seem to relish killing animals so I'd be surprised if ancient hunters had more sensitive morals surrounding killing. It is generally thought that many deities with totem animals or animal heads evolved from the spiritual shamanic connections we have with these particular animals. And so if a human sacrifice cannot be offered up in honour of a deity then an animal can instead. So for Hekate you'd expect a dog sacrifice, with Bacchus a bull and so on.

The wish people had to please and appease and be forgiven for killing were a prime motivation. At a basic level this makes perfect sense — when we wish to please someone, we show them love and respect and gift them. There is little or no difference in how our pagan ancestors related to the divine. And so it also follows that the greater the need the greater the sacrifice.

Evidence of human sacrifice has been found in virtually every ancient culture all over the world. It is the ultimate gift to a deity, the giving of a life. But the original reasons for it seem obscure. There seem to be many. Some used it to help groups overcome the fears associated with facing great mass unknowns. These could be starvation, drought, some sort of environmental catastrophe, anything where the priests or shamans were faced with group terror. It isn't such a massive leap to go from killing people in war to offering their lives up to a God or Goddess. The consuming of human sacrifices also seems evident in some cultures. It is often found that the eating of the flesh is seen as a sign of respect for the life spent. There cannot be anything quite so important as the giving of a life. To actually kill an animal or person in cold blood merely to be offered up to a God or Goddess is the ultimate sacrifice.

There seems a clear distinction between animal sacrifices that continued long after most cultures had abandoned human sacrifices and ritual killings. Ritual killings were often of prisoners of war or punishments for crimes. Some might have offered them up to deities and some might just have been for the benefit of the ruler to enforce his rules by publically demonstrating his power. But human sacrifices to deities were often slightly different affairs, and carried out in a more stylised format, often *in* a religious structure or *on* one. They were still conducted in front of an audience but the emphasis was on the care and respect shown to the sacrifice and the importance of it to those who offered it up.

Anatolia

It's not known for sure what came first, animal or human sacrifice. The earliest temple structure found to date is in southern Turkey at Gobekli Tepe. Thought to be 12,000 years old, it pre-dates our previous evidence for farming and settling. There are human remains and most of them seem to be decapitated. This might be pre or post death. Human sacrifice hasn't been confirmed as having taken place here but it hasn't been discounted either. It is agreed among most scholars including the head of archaeology Klaus Schmidt, that a death cult of some sort began here. Whether it was of a simply shamanic ancestral variety or a more sacrificial sort is not known for sure as yet. But with the majority of the site still to be excavated it might well throw up a few more surprises yet.

Early Hebrew

It is certain that many tribes practiced human sacrifice in early Judaism but considering most of them had roots in earlier pagan traditions in the Middle East it is not surprising. Jericho is about 9,000 years old and Hiel buried nine of his sons under its walls. The Old Testament is full of examples of human sacrifice. Abraham, the legendary founder of the Hebrew peoples, was also prepared to make a sacrifice to this God who demanded his first born 'promised son', Isaac, as an offering to him. Abraham has a dream in which he is instructed by God to take his son to the temple and offer him up. What is most surprising is that Isaac agrees to it. Now Isaac was not the only son of Abraham's but his only by his wife Sarah. He had an older son Ishmael who was born of a surrogate mother. Abraham does as he is told and takes Isaac to the altar. He is about to slit the child's throat when an angel, we don't know which one, intervenes and says Abraham has done all he needs to do and that a ram can be sacrificed instead of Isaac.

This recount of a near human sacrifice is typical of extremist religious fervour. All the Abrahamic religions, and branches thereof, have this story underlying their faith but it is one many today are not overly comfortable with. Seeing the Hebrew, Christian and Islamic Godhead as a bloodthirsty deity, keen to see how far his believers will go for the love of their God, is an attitude still current today, and while few animals are now sacrificed in place of people, many people are still being sacrificed in the name of this God by all manner of fundamentalists.

Greek & Roman

It is fair to say that we have evidence going back at least 9,000 years that human sacrifice and religion have gone hand in hand. Indeed it wasn't until 97 BCE that Rome banned human sacrifice. Romans often sacrificed prisoners of war and criminals but there's wasn't always a bloody affair as they often liked to bury such sacrifices alive, so these weren't religious rites as such. They certainly practised human blood sports, as the gladiator tradition testifies to, and this continued well after the ban of human sacrifices. It seems that sport was excluded from such laws, and they definitely killed early Christians before their conversion. Young lads were offered up to the Goddess Mania, but their main blood sacrifice came with animal donations.

Human Sacrifices

Although Greek mythology tells of human sacrifice, they also tended to stick to animal sacrifice rather than human for the most part. This might come as a surprise but the only exception is Sparta, where they did indulge in ritual human sacrifice, mainly of prisoners of war. Spartans also practiced flagellation as a form of blood sacrifice, usually to Artemis. The few human sacrifices that did occur usually ended up with the carcass being thrown into the sea after the ritual.

Egypt

Evidence of human sacrifice in Egypt is thin on the ground. It definitely occurred but, as in Greece, it wasn't very common. There are grounds to believe it happened from the first dynasty and then, aside from the times of great famines causing cannibalism, it faded from popularity, with particular animal sacrifices taking its place.

The God Shezmu is a bloody character who encourages cannibalism. The Pharaoh Unas who reigned in 2350 BCE endorsed the killing and consuming of people of all ages, from infants to adults. Apparently he would eat babies in the morning, adults in afternoon and the elderly in the evening. This, however, was fairly unique for Egyptians.

During the time of King Aha and Djer, images of men being ritually killed have been found. It isn't clear whether these were ritualistic sacrifices or mass killings of prisoners and criminals.

Kings and Pharoahs often had their slaves and servants go with them into their tombs or pyramids. This might have been due to the King wishing to make sure he had enough servants in the afterlife. They were rarely killed instantly and often had a pitiful last few days of their lives. More often than not entombed sacrifices were either left to die of thirst or poisoned. They definitely carried on ritually killing prisoners of war but any human sacrifices were over by the time of the Old Kingdom.

The drought and famine of 1201 BCE is well documented. The horror of the poorest people turning to eating their own infants and babies is testified to. Many examples of babies being stolen for food is also accounted. People found doing this were breaking the religious and political laws of the time and were punished for it. There is some art depicting these dreadful times and scenes. The richer people could afford the increase in price of stored grain but the less well off were dying of starvation. This wasn't a blood sacrifice as such, but still the innocent were sacrificed, whether they wanted it or not.

Tibet

It is also a surprise to some to hear that pre-Buddhist Tibet also practised human sacrifice, and there is much evidence of a death cult which included cannibalism. Robert Ekvall, an American anthropologist, discovered evidence of human sacrifice high up in the more remote parts of the Himalayas back in the 1950's. There have also been bodies of babies and children found that are believed to be victims of sacrifice back in the early twentieth century. Animal sacrifice replaced this and auto-bloodletting replaced the animals. But some people were still practising blood rituals there until relatively recently. Considering Tibet is the home of the lamas, and now very much a Buddhist country, this comes as a surprise to many people.

Druids and Celts

The ancient Celtic peoples once shared a culture and language that covered most of Gaul (or France), the British Isles and other parts of Celtic Europe, reaching their height in the Iron Age. Their spiritual priesthood was the Druids. Little is known about these mysterious and magical men. That they held great respect and power is recorded by all written accounts. Their spiritual link with oak and mistletoe is also written about by Pliny the Elder,

Human Sacrifices

and it is also recorded, by Romans visiting our lands, that they most definitely practised regular animal and human sacrifice to their Gods. But this might have been Roman propaganda of the time. Julius Caesar a recorded some of these activities and aimed to convert the Celts to a more Roman way of thinking; he might well have witnessed the origins of the Wicker Man. Here he quotes:

All the people of Gaul are completely devoted to religion, and for this reason those who are greatly affected by diseases and in the dangers of battle either sacrifice human victims or vow to do so using the Druids as administrators to these sacrifices, since it is judged that unless for a man's life a man's life is given back, the will of the immortal gods cannot be placated. In public affairs they have instituted the same kind of sacrifice. Others have effigies of great size interwoven with twigs, the limbs of which are filled up with living people which are set on fire from below, and the people are deprived of life surrounded by flames. It is judged that the punishment of those who participated in theft or brigandage or other crimes are more pleasing to the immortal gods; but when the supplies of this kind fail, they even go so low as to inflict punishment on the innocent. (15 March, 44 BCE. *De Bello Gallico* 6.16).

This paints a different picture from the white-robed solemn Bards and Ovates of the modern neo-druidic path, whose only offerings are of the non-blood varieties, but there is still very little proof that these reports are accurate or definitive in any way. That they existed is true. And that they were the ruling priestly elite is also highly likely. The very word Druid comes from the Welsh word *dryw*, meaning 'seer', and they were also known for their sorcery and magical abilities. They also seem to have had many shamanic qualities, as related by Diodorus Siculus, who said that they were able to 'read' the activities of animals and birds and divine from them. The bulk of their rituals etc. seemed to take place in woodland and/or caves. Some Gods were only able to be contacted through Druidic magic, so they were often seen as being on a par with nobility in status, and were not expected to go to war or fight. It was Julius Caesar who wrote of the Wicker Man and told of how a large wooden effigy of a man would be created that was big enough to contain a living person. He says that it would be done on the instruction of Druids, who used it to burn a human sacrifice, mostly male criminal types, but not always.

Another way in which Romans reported that Druid sacrifices took place was on stone slabs with a ritual knife straight to the heart of the victim, whereupon they would divine information and read into the death throes and contortions of the person's dying agonies. This act of ritual death divination also extended to the reading of entrails of both people and animals. But again we must remember that these are the accounts of Roman invaders to our shores keen to overthrow the Druidic class and impose their own Roman paganism upon us.

The earliest written words on the Druids discovered thus far go back to around 200 BCE but they were thought to be all but wiped out by 200 AD. The Druids themselves had an essentially oral tradition and rarely if ever wrote anything down. The Romans also reported that it would take up to twenty years for an initiate Druid to learn all the songs, stories, myths and legends that contained the spiritual wisdom of his priesthood. It is also interesting to note that they are alleged to have had belief in reincarnation. This might be seen to be at odds with the chances of holding blood sacrifices, for how can such a priesthood carry out such things without also taking a chance of being potentially 'punished' in some way in the next life? If the little remnants of information concerning them are in any way correct, we have a ruling priestly elite with shamanic roots. They are thought to have polytheistic beliefs and held spiritual control over parts of mainland Europe, especially France, all of mainland Britain and

Ireland. They practised magic and sorcery and possibly blood sacrifices up until around 200 AD — how long before that is anyone's guess but definitely in the Iron Age and possibly as far back as the Bronze Age.

The Roman author and naturalist Pliny the Elder is the first to write on the Oak and Misteltoe ritual which also, according to his account, has a sacrificial blood rite incorporated into it. He states:

The druids – that is what they call their magicians – hold nothing more sacred than the mistletoe and a tree on which it is growing, provided it is Valonia Oak Mistletoe is rare and when found it is gathered with great ceremony, and particularly on the sixth day of the moon. Hailing the moon in a native word that means 'healing all things,' they prepare a ritual sacrifice and banquet beneath a tree and bring up two white bulls, whose horns are bound for the first time on this occasion. A priest arrayed in white vestments climbs the tree and, with a golden sickle, cuts down the mistletoe, which is caught in a white cloak. Then finally they kill the victims, praying to a god to render his gift propitious to those on whom he has bestowed it. They believe that mistletoe given in drink will impart fertility to any animal that is barren and that it is an antidote to all poisons

This written witnessed report of an actual Druidic rite is one very few. But whether it is entirely accurate or not we shall never know. We can see some elements that do ring true, however. The ancient Celtic peoples did indeed view the oak as especially sacred. Any miraculous or weird plant was often viewed by our ancestors as particularly gifted from Gods/Goddesses and mistletoe was no exception. It was famous for its medicinal properties. The mistletoe was useful for various things including fertility problems, cancers and insomnia. Both Hippocrates and the 17th-century herbalist Culpepper prescribed it for disorders of the spleen. However, it was also used for epilepsy. Because of its ability to increase uterine contractions Native Americans used it to induce abortion and stimulate contractions during childbirth. Therefore it is not safe to give to a pregnant woman if she wishes to remain that way. In Norse mythology, mistletoe is the only plant that Frigg believes can kill her son. This information is used by Loki who makes a dart from a twig of mistletoe and kills Balder with it. So, it transpires that whether a plant of healing or death, it has connections with both cycles of life in our pagan past. Many Green Man images could well be linked directly with the Druids as they are often of oak leaves and mistletoe. But getting back to Pliny's statement, there are other links with Celtic tradition that have elements of fact corroborated by archaeological evidence. The Celts did indeed leave images of elaborate feasts including bulls and the crescent or waning moon in some Cheiftains tombs such as the Hallstat tomb in Hochdorf. The mention by Pliny of the sixth day of the moon would pertain to the sixth day after the full moon which would make it the waning crescent a time associated with the ridding of things unwanted. This is why modern pagans use this time for healing work and clearing or cleansing rituals.

The sacrificing of sacred bulls also appears on the Gundestrup Cauldron which is thought to have been made at some point during the first century AD. Bull or cattle sacrifice was common all over the world and my speculative explanation for this might be incredibly simple. The most important bovine was the cow. She not only gives birth to more of her own but gives milk as well, and has therefore always been of greater use to us in the West than a provider of mere meat. The beef bullocks are manageable, more or less, when young but only the best are worth allowing to maturity to ensure strong genes are passed on down. So the bulk of our ancestors' beef probably came from young bullocks. The fact that it is specifically white bulls that are mentioned again, makes sense. The oldest breed of cattle known to our shores is White Park Cattle. These ancient bovines were especially revered in Ireland where they were used as a source of currency. So to have ritual sacrifices of these highly regarded bullocks or bulls is not that surprising. The mythological 'bull sleep' ritual otherwise known as Tarbhfless from Ireland was a druidic practise. A specially chosen person, usually a man, would be fed on the flesh of a bull and then chanted on as he went to sleep by no less than four Druid priests. Their aim was to induce a dream that would predict who the next in line for the title of High King of Ireland would be. If successful the information would be taken seriously and acted upon. Here we see further evidence of how important the Druid priesthood were and how much influence they had over a vast number of people covering a huge area and several countries.

In Gallic Blood Rites, in an article written in 2001, Jean-Louis Brunaux writes:

Excavations of sanctuaries in northern France support ancient literary accounts of violent Gallic rituals.

Modern historians, relying on reports by Caesar and others, have characterized the religion of the Celts in Gaul as spontaneous rites, in contrast to the well-planned cultic practices of the Greeks and Romans. Archaeologists have now revealed that the Gauls did, in fact, build permanent ritual sites at places like Gournay sur-Aronde and Ribemont-sur-Ancre in northern France. Dated to the end of the fourth or beginning of the third century BC, these cult centers were the work of warlike tribes called the Belgae, thought to have arrived in northern Gaul from central Europe at the end of the great Celtic invasions of the fourth century BC. The rituals performed at Gournay-sur-Aronde and Ribemont-sur-Ancre, however, went well beyond animal sacrifice, a commonplace rite among the Greeks and Romans, and included the triumphant display of the remains of enemies killed in battle or sacrificed to the gods of the underworld, from whom the Gauls believed they were descended.

Jean-Louis Brunaux directs excavations at Ribemont-sur-Ancre and is the author of Les Religions Galoises (Paris: Editions Errance, 1996).

Another example of possible evidence of human sacrifice is presented in the well-known case of the Lindow Man. Found in 1984 in a peat bog in Cheshire, North West England, he presents archaeologists and historians with a complex dilemma. Because of the well-preserved condition of the body it has been possible to put his age at death as around 25 years. His fingernails are manicured, his hair tidied, his beard trimmed and his teeth in good condition, with no obvious signs of serious disease or illness, all virtues of a man of wealth who perhaps didn't have to undertake any manual labour in his life. He was found buried naked with nothing more than a fox fur armband, so no other evidence of his status is indicated by his clothing or jewellery. That he was 'overkilled' is not in dispute: his head has a massive hole in it, thought by the indentation to have been caused by an axe, and it looks as if there were two of these strikes to his cranium. His back has broken ribs, so he might have been kicked or hit by something, and a thin cord around his throat shows he might well have been strangled.

Archaeologists John Hodgson and Mark Brennand think this might be a ritual sacrificial murder. That it was illegal is also an issue, for we were under Roman rule at the time and they had outlawed human sacrifice. Historian Ronald Hutton is not convinced that this is evidence of a druidic sacrifice, however. Excessive copper content in his body might be indicative of his body being painted before he was killed, which again suggests ritual, but this is not verified or confirmed. It is also possible that if he were rich he was murdered, but why go to such lengths? It might explain his nakedness but he might also have been stripped of his clothing to humiliate him, and killed ritualistically for some heinous crime to the local community, but it also follows that his attire might have been worth selling by thieves. The jury is out on Lindow man but if you are interested, his remains can be viewed in the British Museum.

Human Sacrifices

Germanic & Norse

The Germanic peoples practised human sacrifice occasionally. There are very few written accounts, but one recorded by Ibn Fadlan tells the story of a slave girl wanting to be buried with her lord and master. The belief that any woman accompanying a man on such a journey would be elevated to his wife in the next world was obviously held strongly by this girl. But it was more specific than that; she hadn't taken into account that it only applied to women throwing themselves on funeral pyres, not burials. This seems related to a lesser extent to Indian funeral pyres where, in some paths and castes it was common until relatively recently for wives to be burnt with their dead husband. The Indian practice of Sati, as it is called, is an entirely different yet similar tradition. The German slave girl however, must have been desperate to improve her lot, and a very devout believer in the myths.

Some believe that there was also a practice of strangulation rituals to Odin. These are unsubstantiated for the most part and although many such bodies have been found, including the well preserved Tolland Man found in a Jutland peat bog, no written accounts of such rituals have as yet been discovered. This doesn't rule it out as having happened though. Some devotees of Odin in that region of Denmark might well have decided that offering up the odd strangled sacrifice was appeasing and appropriate.

The Germanic and Norse men and women tended to hold their spiritual rituals outside in groves and on hills or places deemed sacred, rather than in temples. But there is at least one exception to this at Uppsala in Sweden. The Heimskringla sagas from Iceland were translated towards the end of the nineteenth century and one such story relates the tale of King Aun who went as far as sacrificing nine of his sons. This might also have an Odinic connection, Odin having hung himself for nine days and nights in order to gain the wisdom of the runes. There was also a tradition of Swedish Kings sacrificing male slaves during Yule every nine years at the Temple of Uppsala. Kings could also be disposed of by their subjects if found wanting, or if the community were suffering hardships and the Kings were failing in their offerings and petitions to their deities. The ruling elite of the Norse and Germanic peoples didn't seem to have the same amount of safety or immunity that many subsequent Anglo-Saxons gained.

Hindu Thuggees

The Hindu Goddess Kali has a long association with blood and death. Although most sacrifices made in her honour are considered legal and involve animals, there was one band of people who took it upon themselves to offer up human sacrifices.

This extreme and debatable example of Kali sacrifice was carried out in her name by Thuggees. These bands of itinerant travellers would deliberately join people making journeys across India and strangle them in their sleep, or when their barriers were down. They then stole whatever they could from their victims. They claimed to be carrying out these crimes in the name of Kali but there is a modern-day viewpoint that this might have been exaggerated by British colonialists. The vast majority of Hindus that worshipped and made offerings to Kali were not Thuggees, however.

Thuggees seem to have evolved an underclass that gained almost a sort of subcultural heroism. Most Thuggees would pass their 'craft,' and I use the term extremely loosely here, to their sons. Outsiders could be enlisted, and some actually chose to be. To those in a lower caste, this criminal activity might have seemed appealing, especially as the bond of blood between Thuggee offered them a certain level of protection. According to Sir H.M. Elliot in his book The History of India, 'In the reign of that sultan [about 1290], some Thugs were taken in Delhi, and a man belonging to that fraternity was the means of about a thousand being captured.

Human Sacrifices

But not one of these did the sultan have killed. He gave orders for them to be put into boats and to be conveyed into the lower country, to the neighborhood of Lakhauti, where they were to be set free. The Thugs would thus have to dwell about Lakhnauti and would not trouble the neighborhood of Delhi any more.'

Occasionally, Thuggees would keep hold of children of murdered travellers to give the illusion to people that they were merely a family group travelling together innocently. Their preferred method of dispatching their sacrifice to Kali was strangulation, which ensured a silent kill. But they often carried out post-mortem atrocities such as boring out eyeballs. Why isn't clear, but if they really did do some of these things in her name then she would have wanted a few drops of blood to fall. The Thuggees claimed they were reenacting Kalis' battle with Raktabija and that was their excuse. The Indian government took a different stance, especially once the British were in rule.

By the 1830s they were eventually all but removed and had been got rid of by William Bentinck and William Henry Sleeman. These two men set out as sheriffs to crack down on these thugs and murderous thieves who gave other Hindus a very bad name. At their height it is estimated by the Guinness Book of Records that they might have been responsible for over 2,000,000 murders but other numbers cite it as being more around the 50,000 mark.

Those who managed to escape or leave the Thuggee tribe to tell the tale said that the murders were always very ritualistic, and they often liked to use wells as places to dispose of the bodies afterwards. They worked as a team, with each person in the Thuggee tribe having a specific job to do. This made them very effective and their ability to deceive was legendary. They would gain the confidence of travellers, and often travel many hundreds of miles with them before killing their desired sacrifice. A remnant of their acts still lives on today in our own language in our use of the word 'thug', even though it now has slightly different emphasis.

Mesoamerica

Of all the peoples throughout history synonymous with human sacrifice, the Aztecs stand out as the bloodiest by far. Most of the information we have about them came from Spaniards whose initial conquest of the Aztec empire took place in 1519-20. The traditions and rituals of the Aztecs shocked and horrified many of the Spanish. When offered food sprinkled with the blood of sacrificed people Cortes was not overly impressed. And yet to turn it down was an insult. The conquest of the major city took a year but the Aztecs, although beaten, still offered up sacrifices.

One place that is synonymous with Aztec bloodlust is Tlateloco. Here Spaniards were greeted by the sight of *tzompantli*, a wall with literally thousands of skulls of sacrificed victims. The bulk of the sacrificed came from the victims of war. The Aztecs were a warrior race. The close bond between rulership, war and sacrifice remained unbroken until 1520 when they were beaten by the superior firepower of the Spanish conquistadors.

The sacrificing of the victims could sometimes go on for days and usually took place at the top of their pyramid temple structures. In one account from Tenochtitlan, a bloody sacrifice went on for so long and killed so many people that rivers of blood were literally cascading down the pyramid steps onto the white marble below.

The Aztec peoples believed that human blood was necessary for the continued fertilisation of the soil. No other blood would do. The underlying purpose of their often elaborate rites and blood sacrifices was to fulfil an obligation to return energy from society to feed the earth, sky and waters. They also considered ritual sacrifices essential for the continuation of the cycle of life and death. Slaves were often offered up as sacrifices and often kept purely for that purpose.

The people also practiced auto-sacrifice and would cut

themselves deliberately or prick their skin to make it bleed. Their primary cutting tool for such things was the obsidian knife. Obsidian can acquire a very sharp razor blade. Ear lobe fraying and tongue and penis piercing also took place in their culture as alternative blood offerings.

Occasionally they would eat the severed limbs and hearts of sacrificed victims during festivals and banquets that often went on for up to a week at a time.

To the invading Spaniards they must have seemed a bloody and primitive race; with the Spanish came Catholicism which was to eventually replace the indigenous beliefs.

Of all the Mesoamerican peoples the Aztecs were by far the bloodiest. The Mayans practised bloodletting and also smeared food with blood. The ruler would voluntarily pierce his penis or tongue and the blood produced would be smeared on the effigies and offerings on an altar, which was then often burned during the ritual. They saw the menstrual blood of the ruling man's wives as highly potent and the best offering for the land. They also held human sacrifice rituals, but not so often as the Aztecs.

The Olmecs left archaeological evidence of blades and perforating tools for bloodletting, but their art doesn't display human sacrifice. It might have occurred, however, as bodies have been found that appear to have been sacrificed.

The Incas had over 12 million people at their height, but they only held onto their empire for a century. They definitely held human sacrifices. Theirs were slightly different to other Mesoamerican nations — they sacrificed children.

The children of the ruling elite were often chosen by the priests or shamans. This was quite a clever move by the spiritual guides of their society. It meant that no one was exempt and power meant sacrifice. Children were taken from the age of six to their teens. The shaman would care for them for several months and feed them well. Then, a few months before they were due to be sacrificed, they began their long climb into the heights of the Andes. The children were often sedated both to help overcome fear and aid them with altitude sickness. Coca leaves were given to them to chew on, and maize beer was offered to them to drink. The children were either left to perish in the icy cold of the mountains or crushed and asphyxiated by strangulation. Their clothing was marked with spiritual symbolism. Food and effigies were often left with them. Their bodies mummified naturally in the cold temperatures and are some of the best preserved of their kind in the world.

One of the first recorded stories of the first Mesoamerican human sacrifice concerns the flaying of the daughter of the king Cóxcox of Culhuacan. What on earth would provoke a king to offer his own daughter? This ultimate act of giving your life or the life of one you love to your deity is something that crops up in many cultures all over the world. The underlying belief that the Gods themselves gave up their physical bodies for the people so that they could live also explains the philosophy behind human sacrifice. If you wish to continue to pay the ultimate homage to such deities, you continue to offer up yourselves to them. This also seems prevalent in Mesoamerica. It was certainly what the Spanish found when they encountered and eventually conquered them. A major core belief is hard to shift, but the Spaniards came with Catholicism at their spiritual helm and it clashed with the native religions in a way they found barbaric and impossible to understand. For although the roots of their book religion had blood all over them, it was an aspect that most of Christianity had moved away from, no longer seeing the spilling of blood as a necessity in ritual context, preferring to spill it through religious wars instead.

The peoples of Mesoamerica were happy to offer up their own lives or the lives of their children to their Gods, they prayed for it to be asked of them as a blessing upon their families. For if you place more importance upon the spiritual link you have with deities than the physical connection you have with your families and friends then the Gods will always win out. They will get their pound of flesh and quart of blood. The priests who took responsibility for choosing who lived and who died had very heavy responsibilities placed upon them.

There is also evidence among the Incas that occasional environmental changes and long-standing droughts caused immense suffering, and it was probably this that made them create the massive stone artworks and lines in the desert. The need to maintain predictable weather patterns became imperative for all settled cultures across the world, and continues to this day. Without regular rain and sun, crops simply don't grow. They did however have at least 18 festival days a year. And it also appears they made human sacrifices on each of these weekends to appease the the Gods.

Native American: The Pawnee

The Pawnee peoples of Northern America had one particular blood sacrifice that tied in with the idea of death and re-birth and was believed to ensure the continued fertility of the crops. The ritual itself might be of interest to modern day Western pagans. It is called The Morning Star ritual. The Pawnee believed that the first ever female was born of the Morning Star or Venus. She was a result of the Morning Star and Evening Star mating. The Morning Star was seen as representing the male energy and the evening the female, as the latter was linked with darkness and mysterious magic. In a way this makes sense. The gestation of a baby happens in the darkness of the mother's womb, and so the two were linked. Naturally we now know that both the Morning Star and Evening Star are one and the same.

The band of the Pawnee that practised the ritual were the Skidi. There are several bands or divisions within the Pawnee peoples that originally split into two major ones: the Northern and Southern tribes. Pawnee was the language of the peoples, as there were many tribes in one, all sharing a similar culture and same tongue. The ritual took place in the autumn and would follow the awaited dream of the Morning Star by a warrior in the tribe. The men were either warriors or hunters but sometimes both. The women grew food, prepared food, made the houses and took care of the children. Spiritual matters were mostly carried out by men. The Skidi of the Pawnee believed that this ritual was essential to guarantee continued fertility and ensure the arrival of spring after the winter months. As they saw the first person born as female, they sacrificed a girl. The girl would not be one of theirs however; they would take a girl from an enemy tribe. The warrior who had the dream would work together with the priest of the tribe to discover by various methods which tribe and which girl to take. Once all the preparations were ready they would steal the girl, a difficult feat in itself and one that would risk war. The girl would be unmarried without children, but she was usually of child bearing age. The ritual itself would take place in early spring so the tribe would care for the girl throughout the winter months as if she were their own.

The ritual was carried out with much emphasis on the relevance of the items used to carry out the sacrifice. A scaffold or pole would be erected in a pit and the pole would be covered in the skins of animals chosen by the priest. Other totemic artefacts such as feathers, skulls, etc. were also attached to the pole.

Once the Morning Star rose with a red hue around it, the priest would know it was time for the ritual. The position of the pole was also important as the Pawnee worked with the four cardinal directions and importance was placed upon the direction of the girl, who would face east. She would be brought out and tied to the pole and an arrow shot into her heart as soon as the Morning Star was visible in the sky. Other braves would then fire more arrows into her to make sure she was properly dead as quickly as possible.

The whole village would attend this ritual, children and infants included. Once the girl was limp and lifeless she would be taken down, the arrows removed and her body faced down on the earth so that her blood could flow into the earth. This being the magic required to bring on spring and aid their fertility. The last known witnessed ritual took place in 1838 on April 22nd. She was a child of 14 known as Haxti who was from the Oglala Lakota tribe. The Missouri Gazette recorded this particular event.

Pressure was put upon the Skidi by other bands of the Pawnee to cease their Morning Star Ritual as the increasingly strong influence of the New Americans arriving on the East Coast meant their ancient barbaric sacrifices could not continue. The whole country was changing at an alarming rate and as land was swallowed up by Europeans so their religion, Christianity mostly, was also being enforced on both their own people and the Native Americans they were encountering. By the mid nineteenth century the old ways were diminishing fast and there was no place for such traditions in the New America that was to follow.

But before we sit in judgment of their practices it helps to remember these traditions were devoutly religious and woven deeply into their spiritual beliefs. The loss of this one life brought new hope and reassurance to the band or village. This might seem, by our standards, an unnecessary death but to the Pawnee it was imperative to the continuation of their well being and fertility.

They weren't alone among Native tribes to practise sacrifice. Those who followed the Sun Dance tradition also had their own sacrificial blood sacrifices.

The Sun Dance is older than the Ghost Dance practiced by the Pawnee. It has many names and is sometimes called the Rain Dance, Medicine Dance or Thirst Dance depending on the tribe carrying it out. The Sun Dance in all its guises is practiced by the Plains Natives. The ritual is held in the spring and like the Morning Star rite it lasts for four days. Participants usually fast prior to the ritual and the dance with its drumming and pipes allows people to go into trance and commune with the spirits of the air, water and earth. These beings are believed to be the most important, second only to the creator or Great Spirit. Many people attend this annual event but non natives are discouraged and even banned now due to a decision taken back in 1997 by the elders of several tribes including Lakota, Cheyenne, Creed, Dakota and Nakota tribes.

During the part of the ritual given to the making of sacred offerings, the tradition was to make literal flesh sacrifices. These were mostly of the animal, rather than the human variety that the Pawnee make, but these days the piercing of skin is considered sufficient to appease the spirits. Men are pierced on their chests and backs whilst women are cut on their arms. Once worked up into an ecstatic trance by the low blood sugar combined with dance, it is unlikely that they felt any pain when being pierced. The resulting scars would be worn with extreme pride because they had been able to offer their own blood to the spirits. Those who give their blood see it as an honour, believing it will improve the hunting and gathering of the future season. In these days it still has relevance depending on how the tribe now earns their living.

Previous forms of flesh sacrifices were outlawed in 1895. This has been largely upheld by most tribes but the piercing of skin does still occur occasionally. It is difficult to say for sure if this is exactly the case for, like so many of these ancient blood sacrifices and offerings, once they are made illegal they tend to go underground. As most tribes are opposed to outsiders taking part ,let alone recording or filming their rituals, we will never know for sure if they still practice within the modern laws or outside of them sometimes.

Papua New Guinea

This part of the world has managed to hit the headlines a few times over the last twenty years or so due to reported incidents of human sacrifice. The cases seem wound up in rumors of sorcery and black magic being spread by Christian cults on the islands. Morobe province is one such place where clashes between leaders of cults and police have occurred as a result of ritual beheadings. It is in the more mountainous regions that these rituals take place and some put it down to the increasing numbers of people dying of AIDS. Some villagers are blaming witchcraft for the disease and this has triggered some of the extreme cases of human sacrifice. Any perceived 'witch' or sorcerer considered responsible for the illness is then beheaded and the head impaled as an example to others. In one such case in the town of Finschafen, a child believed to be a witch was kidnapped and police had a prolonged chase that involved gunfire to try and save the youngster. Paranoia seems at the root of many of the killings, with a lack of true understanding also playing a large part between tribes and their beliefs. With extremist Christian cults on one side and forms of tribal voodoo-style practices on the other, clashes sadly seem inevitable.

Human Muti Killings

This form of sacrifice occurs mainly in Nigeria and South Africa and is practiced by a small minority of Umthakathi, or those who have the title of witches. This isn't thought to be rooted in an ancient traditional practice and seems more modern than many people may believe it to be. These paid magical assassins ritualistically murder children and adults whilst others chant, clap and dance. While he is dismembering the still-living sacrifice the witchdoctor will aim, with assistance of the spirit realm, to send the life force of the person concerned into one or two limbs or body parts before they die. The person is also often tortured beforehand. Why they do this isn't clear, and is probably more for fear-inducing effect and/or sadistic enjoyment than any magical reason. These body parts are believed to then contain the life force of the person and are worth a great deal on the black market. It is believed a human muti ceremony can give the parts enough magical power to bring whoever buys them great riches and power.

Human muti is a growing problem in Africa. Muti in itself means medicine. Not all Umthakathi practise sacrificial human muti as most stick to ancestral worship and more traditional herbal medicine, but human muti killing is big money, and is therefore very tempting to those lacking much in the way of ethics and morals who have many hungry mouths to feed. Most traditional muti practitioners look down on this variety of muti, but are not averse to occasional animal muti.

Back in 2001 Thames Police were alerted to the torso of a child floating down the river. Nicknamed 'Adam', the boy was thought to have been between 5 and 7 years old. His head and limbs had all been removed, along with his penis. This echoed a similar finding back in 1969 of a baby girl found in similar circumstances. One extra, and peculiar, thing was that the boy's orange shorts had been put back on after the mutilation. On examining the torso it was found that whoever killed him knew what they were doing. The job had been done with the skills of a butcher. He had, only recently, been eating Western food and forensic examination concluded that he had only been in the country for about a week. DNA results placed his home firmly in Nigeria and narrowed it down to between two towns. Advice was sought from various voodoo practitioners and experts in their field, who backed up the growing suspicions that this was the results of a kill-to-order human muti ritual. They affirmed that the boy would have been sedated and strangled just before his throat was cut and some of his blood drained for ritual consumption. His penis and eyes would have been preserved in spirit for future use. He was decapitated as his head represented his intelligence and independence, and his limbs removed as they were symbolic of his creativity and mobility.

After making a trip to Africa, the detectives investigating this case faced the unpleasant fact that this kind of behaviour is commonplace; an estimated 300-plus killings associated with deliberate muti take place each year. The body parts are worth much money on the black market. This particular offering was thought to have been made to the God Oshun. Oshun has the colour orange associated with him, alongside eternal life. He is also a water deity with a river named after him. These associations explained the torso being thrown into the Thames and the replacing of the orange shorts.

Journalist Jimmy Lee Shrive writes extensively on this case in his book Blood Rites, and even talked with Scotland Yard about it. He wanted to know why they were so convinced that this was a human sacrifice and involved black magic. He also wanted to know if other more conventional reasons for the child having been killed had been explored, such as straightforward murder or the possible work of a murdering paedophile. They assured him all avenues had been looked into and the bulk of the evidence still led them to think it was the darker side of voodoo.

It must also be noted here that the vast majority of voodoo practitioners don't deal in the remains of murdered victims, nor do they practice human muti killings. Like every form of religion, voodoo has a darker side and there are always those who will abuse the power and knowledge to urge spirits to do evil works.

As a final, and quite reassuring balance, Jimmy Lee Shrive sought the assistance of a Native American spirit doctor Crazywolf from the Ojibwa tribe. He visited London and made contact with Adam's soul. He said that although a Christian burial had taken place for the boy, it didn't make any difference to the fact that Adam's soul was still in the hands of evil spirits conjured for the benefits of those who killed him. His opinion was that Adam's was a drug-related killing by drug traffickers who were keen to use black magic to aid them in their illegal work. Together, Jimmy and Crazywolf performed a ritual to release Adam's soul and send it on to the otherworld.

Sacrifices seem to operate on a sliding scale. A very poor man offering his last penny to buy a dove to sacrifice might gain more than a rich man offering the same beast; it all seems relative. It isn't always a case of the larger the sacrifice the greater the spiritual return. But whether it be for the cleansing of sins, enhancing lives in other ways or giving thanks, all sacrifices are made with one solitary purpose: gain. Through making the sacrifice one hopes to gain in another direction. The act of taking a life being the greatest sacrifice anyone can make, with human sacrifice being the highest of all.

Human sacrifices were made by our pagan ancestors for a variety of reasons. Some were a reaction to environmental disasters in an attempt to appease whichever deity they felt caused the problem. Some were the result of enforced cannibalism due to starvation. In other cases they were simply honouring the spiritual memory of the living God or Goddess. Many were to mark the building of temples and undertaken in order to give the greatest offering thought possible to the deity whose religious building it was constructed in honour and worship of. There were human sacrifices to mark the passing of a leader to accompany them on their journey. Many pharaohs had people sealed shut inside pyramids and tombs to join the King or Queen in the afterlife. And some were made prior to a battle or war. There is evidence all over the world for human and animal sacrifices. From the bones, alone archaeologists are able to determine how the person or animal died. And some marks are most obviously sacrificial and often pre-date our written history by many thousands of years. Sacrifices were often made voluntarily and seen in many cultures, like the Inca's for example, as an honour and blessing upon the family. If your belief system is so deeply entrenched in your psyche that you can say you know that the sacrificed child or adult will ascend to the Gods, and the spirit of this person will be elevated to a higher state of being, then you accept the necessity more readily.

Human Sacrifices

    This act of offering up the life source of an animal or human being to a deity is practised among some groups of people to this day. We might have more tolerance for animal sacrifices but the vast majority of cultures have moved beyond taking human life in this manner. Religious or spiritual activities or rituals are normally executed for specific purposes or to celebrate the festival of a particular deity or time of year.

Ritual to Invoke Kali

Kali is one aspect of the Mother Goddess of Hinduism.

The darkness associated with her represents the ability of all colours to become invisible when night falls. This lack of colour is often seen as being devoid of distraction, enabling her to transcend this plane. She is liberated from any garb and therefore free of illusion. Her way is truth. She can work karma and set people free from it as represented by the seven hands around her waist. The severed heads are meant to represent the fifty Sanskrit letters. Her right hand represents her creative side, and her left hand the destructive half. She has three eyes representing the past, present and future. These are also seen as the sun, the moon and fire. Her red tongue is not afraid to either say or taste anything.

She is a goddess of powerful transformation of consciousness through death of attachments and ego and acceptance of death in the cycle of life.

It is easy to perform a simple ritual to invoke Kali but you need a reason or intent to do so. Maybe you wish Kali to set you free from a karmic cycle. Perhaps you wish her to help you come to terms with losing a loved one. Or perhaps you wish greater wisdom and enlightenment and the ability to release more love from your heart?

Kali resides in the heart chakra and therefore it is most likely here that you will feel her presence most. You don't have to be Hindu or an initiate, for Kali sees all people as her children. She is a force of nature made manifest for us to connect with and understand.

If you are a Hindu living in Calcutta, her main temple is here, and you'd be sacrificing a goat in her honour. But as it is more likely that you are not, then maybe offering up some food made especially for her will be an alternative. I can't find any examples of rituals that include offering Kali your own blood but this doesn't mean to say you can't. This I leave to your discretion but I suggest including it as a sprinkle offering to go over the food offering.

Another option is to use two candles, one black and one red.

Skulls, hands and flowers might all be good things to represent on your altar to her as will be a centre piece effigy or image of her. You could also have a blue altar cloth to represent Shiva, her consort.

Incense of your own choosing is great and many Indian kinds are quite pungent and sweet champa types.

Naturally being able to activate all your main seven chakras will help increase your connection.

The Calling

I call upon the Great Mother Goddess Kali Durga

Kali the warrior, Kali the destroyer, Kali the opener of the way of light and truth.

She who will free me from karma, she who will rid me of all I've outgrown, she who is within me and protects me from harm, Kali Om Ma, Kali Om Ma.

Oh terrifying Durga who defeats evil and brings life to the pure, who allows death and destruction to have their way as necessity for new life to spring from, she who sees all and knows all, Kali Om Ma, Kali Om Ma.

Help me be at one with your heart and let mine beat to a better rhythm, aid me in my trials and quests and goals, help me overcome my failures and understand better my own mortality, set me free from the restrictions of my ego here tonight that I may see the light hidden in your infinite darkness, Kali Om Ma, Kali Om Ma.

Oh Kali Om Ma
Oh Kail Om Ma
Oh Kali Om Ma
Accept these my offerings to you. (Make offering of food with your own blood sprinkled on it)

Open my heart and seat of true vision
Through your tongue taste my words and know they are true, speak to me of things I need to know, help me accept your wisdom and your love and your protection.
With your left hand destroy that which needs to be destroyed.
With your right hand create that which needs to be created.
Om Kali ma Om Kali ma Om Kali Ma…… (continue chanting this mantra until she arrives).

Once communion is done, thank her and bid her farewell.

CHAPTER 6
Religious Blood Rituals

As I mention in an opening declaration of this book, 'Religion was born of blood and has been steeped in blood ever since.' Name an organised religion and blood sacrifices will have either been a part of their history or are still very much a part of their continued tradition. From Hinduism to the Aztecs to modern day Christianity, and many more besides, blood sacrifices of either animal or human or both are a part of their history. The main reason, seems to an outsider, to be due to the need to appease angry Gods or spirits, but it isn't that simple. One look at the origins of Vodhun or Voodoo will give insight to a deeper blood bond between human and spiritual beings whether they be deities or ancestors. If you count Creole Vodou and Santeria as partly Catholic then these traditions also give regular blood sacrifices, albeit mostly of livestock, and are definitely blended in strongly with Christianity.

For a tradition to evolve and drop some ritual practices is very much the choice of that religion, and often ties in with the politics and changing morals and ethics of the cultures concerned. There are also those who like to give their own blood occasionally to their deities and there are some who follow, like Christians, a symbolic blood sacrifice.

It seems that as the hunting and gathering of Neolithic man became more sophisticated so habits, rituals and wisdom increased regarding each particular animal sought. The sacredness placed upon the hunt was the beginning of deliberate ritualistic blood sacrifices. Sharing the spoils of the day or night was commonplace and each tribe or family group would do so. But there is also much evidence among the vast majority of pre-historic communities that seasonal group gatherings also took place. And it is at these that the first blood sacrifices were most likely made. Sacrificing an animal for a shared feast whilst giving thanks to the spirit of it gels people together it binds them to the blood of the beast. It is well known that many early tribes believed that in consuming any animal you took on its spirit and essence. This primitive, we are what we eat, belief system is literal in its purity but still applies today. And though we rarely consider this when we tuck into our Sunday roast, in some respects it holds true.

It makes sense that the earliest deliberate ritualistic sacrifices were made for group celebrations of one sort or another. It also follows that gratitude for a successful hunt and/or harvest probably comes a close second. But with the creation of farming and ownership of fertile land came a completely new relationship with the earth and mother nature. Now we sought to become creationists ourselves, by attempting to gain mastery over crops and selective breeding of domesticated animals. We had property and land to protect. Protection rituals probably already existed, but had to be altered and expanded upon to account for this new way of life.

Gods were seen in many cultures to reside in high places such as the heavens and mountains. This seems to be the main reason for creating high altars in temples, pyramids and eventually cathedrals. By creating ritual, the priest can impress and mystify his audience from on high or in an inner sanctum. Being able to look down on the masses was popular in some emerging cultures. All manner of props could be utilised from specific ritual knives kept purely for spiritual occasions to elaborate clothing and dance and music all bringing the event alive with potential death. The sacrificial element to the ritual could vary considerably. A lot depended on the type of ritual being held, what for and whether the sacrifice was animal or human. For some it was the climax of the ritual, especially if it was to be a mass human sacrifice. For others it was minimalized, still deemed necessary, but not the main event.

Elements common to many varying cultures and blood rituals include the altar, a ritual knife, incense, food offerings, liquor and sacred vessels, fire and/or candles or lamps, ornate dress for the presiding priesthood and highly prized decoration both for the altar. Also, the accoutrements on it were often made of gold, silver and precious jewels. The ritual knife would be considered sacred and kept separate from other knives and often made from different material to domestic ones. Obsidian was a favourite among the Aztecs and many other peoples around the world as a material to create knives from. It can be fashioned into sharper blades than flint and is not so prolific a resource so was often chosen for ritual purpose prior to metals. By creating glamour early priests and priestesses from many differing cultures set themselves apart from the masses. Their appearance took on an other worldly look. They became exclusive and special.

Although this is generalising, it is true to say that once early civilisations had created their places of worship they had set the scene for the theatrical stage of organised ritual and sacrifice. The rustic, simple shaman was about to enter a new era: the era of performances. And this time demanded drama. Much drama, incredible effort went into many of the rituals. Both from the infrastructure to the other often complex requirements, greater detail was considered and given consideration to. The offering of the sacrifice(s), was often a tiny part of the occasion which frequently took place, and still does, at the end of the ritual or after it. And in nearly all cases and across pretty much all cultures ,the meat was consumed afterwards. To waste the remains of the animal was considered sacrilege.

It is also possible that hallucinogens played a part in ritual sacrifices. Many of the countries that have a history of it also have access to plant-based drugs. From the liberty caps ingested by Celts to the fly agaric of the Norse and Germanic men and women to the peyote cactus of middle and south America and the cannabis of the Middle East and India, our ancestors had many options to choose from. Even the humble rye grass has such properties if allowed to ferment and go mouldy and it was ergot that gave birth to LSD. Anyone who has taken hallucinogens will agree that they alter and enhance our perceptions. They also seem to lower our moral boundaries. Such drugs would be used not only for trance and other world journeys by shamans but might also have been very useful to take during a ritual, especially one involving the taking of a life or blood.

Hebrew

When Jesus the Nazarene arrived in Jerusalem for Passover he lost his temper and turned the tables of the money lenders outside the temple. It was at those specifically touting for sacrificial business that he aimed his attention. The money lenders would place temptation under the noses of the poor, the troubled, the guilt ridden and the desperate. Many were sick or blamed their sins for their ills. Money could be obtained to buy either a dove, goat, sheep or bullock to offer to the temple and the person, though now in debt, would be able to clear his sins away. It infuriated him that 'his father's house' had become a place of thieves. He particularly aimed his fury at the ones selling doves as he knew these were the cheapest offerings and often the ones bought by the poorest people.

Religious Blood Rituals

There is no doubt among biblical scholars that the God of the Hebrew peoples, Yahweh, liked his blood sacrifices. The Old Testament is littered with examples. From the first offering of the sacrificial lamb Abel gives to Yahweh, to Abraham being expected to give his son's life, to the scapegoat on the Day of Atonement being sent out to Azaz-el, blood sacrifices were still popular until long after the time of Christ. The Hebrew peoples offered live sacrifices as well as burnt ones and blood offerings in their temples. The practice most heard of is the Day of Atonement when three sacrifices are made. This ancient practice originated with Aaron and we find it in the Old Testament in Leviticus starting at Verse 6:

6 And Aaron shall present the bullock of the sin-offering, which is for himself, and make atonement for himself, and for his house.

7 And he shall take the two goats, and set them before the LORD at the door of the tent of meeting.

8 And Aaron shall cast lots upon the two goats: one lot for the LORD, and the other lot for Azaz-el.

9 And Aaron shall present the goat upon which the lot fell for the LORD, and offer him for a sin offering.

10 But the goat, on which the lot fell for Azaz-el, shall be set alive before the LORD, to make atonement over him, to send him away for Azaz-el into the wilderness.

11 And Aaron shall present the bullock of the sin-offering, which is for himself, and shall make atonement for himself, and for his house, and shall kill the bullock of the sin-offering which is for himself.

12 And he shall take a censer full of coals of fire from off the altar before the LORD, and his hands full of sweet incense beaten small, and bring it within the veil.

13 And he shall put the incense upon the fire before the LORD, that the cloud of the incense may cover the ark-cover that is upon the testimony, that he die not.

14 And he shall take of the blood of the bullock, and sprinkle it with his finger upon the ark-cover on the east; and before the ark-cover shall he sprinkle of the blood with his finger seven times.

15 Then shall he kill the goat of the sin-offering, that is for the people, and bring his blood within the veil, and do with his blood as he did with the blood of the bullock, and sprinkle it upon the ark-cover, and before the ark-cover.

16 And he shall make atonement for the holy place, because of the uncleannesses of the children of Israel, and because of their transgressions, even all their sins; and so shall he do for the tent of meeting, that dwelleth with them in the midst of their uncleannesses.

17 And there shall be no man in the tent of meeting when he goeth in to make atonement in the holy place, until he come out, and have made atonement for himself, and for his household, and for all the assembly of Israel.

18 And he shall go out unto the altar that is before the LORD, and make atonement for it; and shall take of the blood of the bullock, and of the blood of the goat, and put it upon the horns of the altar round about.

19 And he shall sprinkle of the blood upon it with his finger seven times, and cleanse it, and hallow it from the uncleannesses of the children of Israel.

20 And when he hath made an end of atoning for the holy place, and the tent of meeting, and the altar, he shall present the live goat.

21 And Aaron shall lay both his hands upon the head of the live goat, and confess over him all the iniquities of the children of Israel, and all their transgressions, even all their sins; and he shall put them upon the head of the goat, and shall send him away by the hand of an appointed man into the wilderness.

22 And the goat shall bear upon him all their iniquities unto a land which is cut off; and he shall let go the goat in the wilderness.

23 And Aaron shall come into the tent of meeting, and shall put off the linen garments, which he put on when he went into the holy place, and shall leave them there.

24 And he shall bathe his flesh in water in a holy place and put on

his other vestments, and come forth, and offer his burnt-offering and the burnt-offering of the people, and make atonement for himself and for the people.

25 And the fat of the sin-offering shall he make smoke upon the altar.

26 And he that letteth go the goat for Azaz-el shall wash his clothes, and bathe his flesh in water, and afterward he may come into the camp.

27 And the bullock of the sin-offering, and the goat of the sin-offering, whose blood was brought in to make atonement in the holy place, shall be carried forth without the camp; and they shall burn in the fire their skins, and their flesh, and their dung.

28 And he that burneth them shall wash his clothes, and bathe his flesh in water, and afterward he may come into the camp.

29 And it shall be a statute for ever unto you: in the seventh month, on the tenth day of the month, ye shall afflict your souls, and shall do no manner of work, the home-born, or the stranger that sojourneth among you.

30 For on this day shall atonement be made for you, to cleanse you; from all your sins shall ye be clean before the LORD.

This in-depth description of exactly how, when and where the animal sacrifices were made is an excellent example of how people had moved from sacrificing animals purely for food to placing a very different spiritual emphasis upon the act. Now the animals are being killed to rid people of sin. And this atonement continues to this day among Hebrew people as Kapparot. On the eve of Yom Kippur it is traditional among some Jewish peoples to swing a chicken or purse of coins over your head three times. Your sins are now taken on by the purse or bird. This offering can then be killed and given to the poor. Selling the notion that you can rid yourself of sin is very appealing to people, and going to the lengths of ritually killing to enable this act certainly means it is a ritual taken very seriously.

There are strict rules concerning the animals that can be sacrificed. They have to be blemish free and healthy. Some are stipulated as having to be of younger stock. Larger animals could be a shared sacrifice between up to seven people, and it is not uncommon for people to have sacrificial syndicates. Specific prayers must be said over the animal before, during and after the sacrifice. Some animals have a special bath or wash or are painted with religious symbolism or certain colours before being killed. All the meat of the sacrifice is shared out afterwards. The meat of the animal is often thought to have extra special spiritual qualities, after being sacrificed in the presence of God.

These early recorded historical sacrifices are all taken from earlier pagan traditions and all stem from the original moment when man went from foraging and scavenging to killing and hunting. The offering in most cases was an act of gratitude, submission and piety to the deity. Yahweh is renowned for his insistence on obedience to him and his laws as laid down by Moses in the Ten Commandments that are placed in The Ark of the Covenant.

One blood sacrifice that we are all familiar with that continues to this day is the circumcision of Hebrew males. This removal of the foreskin of the male child's penis is normally carried out by a Rabbi before the child is two weeks old, and is believed to have stemmed from Egyptian practices. There is evidence of it on wall art in ancient Egypt. This is not surprising as the ancient Egyptians were pioneers in all sorts of surgery, and though it is thought to be done purely for religious purposes, it is entirely possible that it stemmed from necessity in some cases and just caught on like a fashion.

The Eucharist

The Eucharist is a blood sacrifice supposedly serving as a constant reminder of the blood of Christ that was spilt before his death, ascension and resurrection. This divergence from the Hebrew path of the time was possibly an attempt by Christ to drop the need for the taking of life and shift the responsibility of sacrifice into the Temples domain. By the creation of the Eucharist it is thrown onto the shoulders of the Christian priests to provide the symbolic sacrifice as represented by the bread and wine. Christ's sacrifice was not only his own mortal life but a desire to put an end to sin sacrifices. This put everyone on the same level and removed the corruption associated with the selling of animals for sacrifice. To take his blood and flesh seems cannibalistic and barbaric but at the simplest spiritual level the bread and wine is meant, as it is ingested, to bring you closer to God. By partaking of this religious ritual through Holy Communion, each person is becoming a part of Christ and God, in theory. The fact Christ allegedly gave his life force, blood and flesh, to save all of us from our sins is relived through the various Christian rituals not least of all in taking communion wine and bread. But why would this remnant of The Last Supper still hold strength over the participants to this day? I presume it is because they believe in it. It seems as simple as that. Whether the blood is literal or symbolic doesn't seem to matter but the fact it is sipped from a chalice does take us deeper into Christ's mysteries. Did he do this merely to keep the physical/spiritual link over the eons? Or has a chunk of the Eucharist been dropped, forgotten, ignored or deliberately missed out for thousands of years? It is entirely possible that it has. The modern Christian description of the Eucharist normally goes like this:

The Eucharist, also called Holy Communion, the Sacrament of the Altar, the Blessed Sacrament, the Lord's Supper, and other names, is a Christian sacrament or ordinance. It is re-inacted in accordance with Jesus' instruction at the Last Supper, as recorded in several books of the New Testament, that his followers do the same in remembrance of Him as he did when he gave his disciples bread, saying, 'This is my body', and gave them wine, saying, 'This is my blood'.

If we look at the two main components of the Eucharist, bread and wine, the bread is traditionally unleavened and the wine red. They are served from a special platter and goblet or chalice. The platter is probably irrelevant, but the chalice is not. Some that say it represents the womb which gives a very different emphasis to the wine. Is it Christ's blood we are partaking of or Mary's menstrual blood? And if so which Mary; his virginal mother, or the Magdalene? Or do the chalice and the wine represent all women and all wombs and, therefore, could Christ be attempting to reinstate the long forgotten Goddess whilst ridding us of animal sacrifice?

It is interesting to try putting ourselves back into the mind set of the times, if that is at all possible. In the time of Christ it was women who made the bread and most of the wine and women who set the table and served these substances to people. Yet even to this day, women are forbidden to give communion. This seems a deliberate act taken to supress the feminine role in the Eucharist. Surely it makes more sense to hand this duty and ritual over to women? It would make more sense this way, unless you wished to exclude the feminine and divert the eyes of future generations towards this being a purely male oriented ritual.

The Eucharist also seems then to be harkening back to the times of blood sacrifices, which were still made during the time of Christ at the Temple in Jerusalem. But if you place a feminine emphasis upon it then it becomes part of an even older spiritual *thanksgiving* (Eucharist in Greek means thanksgiving): that of the sacrifice all women make giving their blood and flesh to create and sustain life.

All current religious Christian bodies that celebrate the Eucharist will say it is the symbolic sacrifice Christ was about to make and definitely concerns *his* blood and *his* flesh as written in the religious books that followed his life, especially The New Testament. But we also know that many of the older knowledge and books were deliberately not included in the final analysis. The hidden books of the Bible have only really come to light over the last 40 years or so, and even though they have been dated, their provenance is still disputed by many, not least the Catholic Church.

The transubstantiation that is meant to occur as one receives Holy Communion is taken seriously by those who partake of it. As it is ingested, so a portion of divinity also manifests within the person. To imbue wine and bread with divine energy is a commonplace event in our pagan past and present. Today pagans all over the world still give offerings to their deities and often these take the form of wine and food. After the ritual is completed the wine and food is ingested by those present as it is deemed magical and spiritually enhanced by the ritual that has taken place. This sacrament is far older than the Eucharist and there are many who today claim the Eucharist does owe it's origins to pagan blood offerings. This could well be true or, at least, where Christ took his inspiration. But if we return to the theory that the chalice does indeed represent the womb then the previously omitted divine feminine is included at the most holy and intimate level. If we then admit that the bread is meant to be representative of the bodies of all women, then it is a celebration of his life as given to him by his mother. It is interesting to note that Christ's inherent divinity is not believed to be a result of his mothers Immaculate Conception but is considered to be a direct gift from God. Mary's assumption of God-given divinity only occurs after her ascension.

The beliefs born of these ancient religious texts are of a time when mankind assumed that a woman in herself was not fertile. This limited sexual reproductive knowledge presumed that the seed was in the man and placed inside the woman. The function of the ovaries didn't seem to be common knowledge at this time in history in the Middle East. Women were merely incubators and the womb a house for the male seed to grow in. Little did they know that all foetuses begin life as female, with sexual dominance only manifesting at a later date. They knew that blood played a part and understood a connection between the monthly bleed and lack of conception, but the Abrahamic paths put paid to this, relegating menstrual blood along with other blood to an unclean and potentially dangerous position. This 'blood shift' is evident on many levels of belief, from the treatment of women to food to habits and practices. Blood was suddenly a very dirty word and yet Christ obviously didn't think so. The fact he chose to reintroduce a sacred aspect to blood right at the end of his life is pertinent. He knew his own life force was about to be drained from him through the wounds of the crucifixion and yet wants his followers to view blood in a positive light. He is trying to re-educate them at the last minute. He wants them to remember his sacrifice every time they partake of the Eucharist but he also leaves enough symbolism to query his true underlying motives, if there were any.

If we now stretch our imaginations to see the blood and flesh of Christ as also representing the menstrual blood and flesh of his mother, it takes on another form. No one can deny that without the one there could not have been the other. Even God needed a mortal woman to incubate and give birth to this divine being. The Catholic Church holds 'Our Lady' in high esteem but never as highly as her son Christ. Her blood was spilt upon a bed of straw to bring him into the world. And yet his relationship with his mother is one of mentor to her and she comes across as a devotee of him. This mother/son relationship is often likened to the Egyptian Goddess Isis and her magically conceived son Horus and many think this is the source of the Christian myth. In this myth Osiris is betrayed and murdered, dies and is resurrected by Isis and her sister Nephthys long enough to conceive Horus. In the Christian myth, Mother Mary made a spiritual and blood sacrifice to bring Christ into the world, as all women do when they have children, and Christ makes an equal sacrifice at the apparent end of his life. For his to be a literal death sacrifice, the resurrection would not have occurred but according to scripture it did and the whole basis of the Christian faith hangs on this miracle. Whether Jesus of Nazereth really died on the cross is also unprovable and debatable but thousands of millions of people all over the world believe he did, and in many cases over the last two thousand years have been prepared to follow his martyrdom and die for this belief. The jury will probably remain out on this subject eternally but even for a pagan like myself it is nonetheless a fascinating subject to consider.

Hinduism

One pagan tradition known for blood sacrifice is Hinduism. Not all deities are given blood, but those who are most strongly linked to it still demand their offerings. One such example is the Goddess Kali. This terrifying and ferocious mother Goddess likes her blood. Her origins lay in the Goddess Durga. But Kali earned her bloody reputation from her battle with evil forces that induced an unbridled blood lust in the Goddess and meant that, in her enthusiasm, she nearly killed everyone. Only Shiva, her consort, was able to stop her by throwing himself in her path. The unexpected sight of her husband pulled her up in her tracks and she responded by sticking her tongue out at him.

She is usually depicted as black with skulls and other bones as her clothing and with no less than four arms. Her eyes are usually bulging giving her a manic appearance. She also holds a sword in one hand and the severed head of a demon in another. As a mother she represents the fiercest aspect of the maternal archetype, a mother who will happily kill. The majority of her temples are found in Eastern India and she often occupies positions close to cremation grounds. Animals are usually killed as quickly and quietly as possible. It is often seen as a bad omen if an animal makes a noise whilst being sacrificed and so the use of hypnotism can often come into play to semi-sedate and relax the animal about to be killed. Sometimes the beast is consumed as part of the ritual and sometimes not.

Other Hindu deities also demand blood spilt in their name, for example in Nepal every 5 years a ritual to the Goddess Gadhimai took place and a staggering 250,000 animals would be sacrificed. This seems a ridiculous amount and it is very hard to believe it really occurred but these are the statistics recorded.

There is even a Hindu religious ritual cockfight that takes place in Bali called Tabuh Rah. This takes place outside a temple, after a long ritual has taken place, and is meant to represent the symbolic act of fighting off evil spirits. The ritual is held to ensure that the ensuing death of the birds, and the spilling of their blood will appease these evil forces and means, in theory, that people will be spared from their worst effects. The cult of the Theyyam Gods are also those for whom ritual cock fighting is linked to.

In more generalized ritual animal sacrifice to some Hindu deities, the method of Jhatka is preferred. This involves of one single blow by axe or sword to decapitate the head of the beast. Other methods such as spikes into hearts and strangulation can also sometimes be utilised. To write about this here in a dispassionate way seems strange. Although I lack personal experience, I know of many people who have travelled to India and witnessed many rites and rituals not practiced in the Western world. Most tend to agree that in context the atmosphere is benevolent and kindness and respect is shown to the animal about to be sacrificed. This often extends to the beast being covered in dye and painted colours associated with the deity it will be giving the life for. The importance of maintaining this practice seems paramount with certain deities, and far less so with others. Many Buddhist influenced paths are against blood rituals. It is not surprising that the path of the vegetarian and vegan spiritualist is somewhat blood free.

Tibet

Tibet was once home to elaborate death rituals. Anyone who has seen a Tibetan ritual skull is impressed with the gilt and decoration and carvings upon it. During the thirteenth century reports came out of Tibet via Mongol sources telling of these rituals. When some elder males of a family died their bodies would be cut up into portions and most of the flesh taken up into the air by vultures and other such carrion. This was symbolic of the angels accepting the body of the dead man. Then the bones were used for all manner of religious and spiritual purposes including the making of musical instruments. The Mongols also say that the head was cooked and consumed by the family, but this wasn't verified or witnessed by any other people and is not considered an absolute truth. It has been confirmed by the Jesuit Father Andrada in 1625 that the skull would then be cleaned and the top of the cranium sliced off. Both parts would then be highly decorated with gold and silver and gems. The skull would then be used for ritual purposes and live on a triangular mount on an altar. The altar was carved with skulls and flames. The skull would be used to pour libation liquor from. It was also common for all deceased male relatives to be treated with the same reverence, minus the eating of the head. The people of Tibet at this time were known as the Isselonians. Some of these practices are thought to be Indian and Russian imports. Once Buddhism replaced the shamanism of the area the blood rituals diminished rapidly.

This ritual use of skulls is found all over the world. Often it is more related to the death of an enemy. Evidence of such skull trophies being made into drinking vessels can be found as tribal customs in Tibet, Scythia (Iran), Turkey, Celtic regions, Germanic areas, Slavonia, Mesoamerica and Australia. The posthumous preservation of skulls is also common in Christianity. Many saints' skulls are kept in cases in cathedrals and churches all over the world. Our word 'cup' originates from Anglo Saxon 'cuppe' meaning skull cap which comes from the German 'kopf'.

The Festival of Ashura — Shi-ite Muslims

It may surprise some of you to know that there are still occasions today during which a blood ritual is carried out by some Shi'ite Muslims, the main one being to honour the day of Ashura. During a ritual called Matam or Malik, held in memory of the martyrdom of the prophet Muhummad's grandson, selective participants go into a special prayer room, bare their chests and deliberately self harm by beating themselves. By the last day of the commemoration this increases in severity to being thrashed on their backs by a bladed scourge called a Zanjeer. The festival also commemorates a battle in which the men were unable to save the life of their leader. Most modern day clerics have dropped the bloody aspect of the rite and only a few still choose to practice it. This painful dedication and devotion to Imam Ali Hussein, the prophet's grandson, takes place in countries such as Iraq, Pakistan, Britain, Kubal, Turkey and India, among others.

Problems arise with this sort of religious rite when children enter into the equation. The ritual can include boys as young as 6 years old and even though it breaks the child protection laws in the UK to flagellate a child, police are reluctant to intervene. It is hard to know if the youngsters have much choice in being a part of the ritual. While one would like to think that they do, it is hard to comprehend a child wishing to be beaten by a whip with sharp blades! I'd like to think this is a very rare occurrence as there are laws to protect young children for a reason. From my own perspective, I wouldn't consider it ethical either to inflict your religious beliefs on your children or to beat them, but this just shows how a massive schism of differing cultural ethics and morals divides people.

Vodhun/Voodoo

This essentially African traditional magical path has migrated to many places around the world and forms of it are found in the Caribbean, Haiti and mainland America among others. Steeped in mystery it has mostly been an oral tradition of initiation, magic and its very name means Garden of Blood and Bones. There are many variations of Voodoo, or Vodhun, and the one we shall briefly explore first is from mainland Africa, in a place called Togo in West Africa. This area has a population of around 4.5 million, many of whom practice traditional Vodhun.

In her book Cord of Blood, Nadia Lovell records her time spent with one of the ethnic groups of the area known as the Watchi who are part of the larger Ewe tribe. The belief that the 'hunka' or cord of blood that connects mother and child extends to the alternate planes of spiritual dimensions abounds in this religion. Therefore, use of blood in ritual and rituals inspired by this blood tie are commonplace. The everyday practical lives of the people and the inner spiritual planes are integrated in a very holistic way. This makes breaking down individual activities and practices a complex task to unravel. Each village will have at least one Vodhun shrine. This is a place declared sacred that is set aside, usually just on the fringes of the village. It will have had a rooting or grounding ritual performed by the one who will be responsible for the shrine, to create the cord between God and man. By seating their deity in a shrine they are able to use it as a focal point and a magical place to make very real connections and hold communions with the deity concerned. The only deity who is not anchored in quite the same way is one known as 'Legba'. This essentially protective spirit is represented outside the shrine.

Hunka stands for 'hun' blood and 'ka' cord. This cord extends into the earth where the blood and bones of the ancestors lie and connect to the living beings today and their individual family ties and ethnic groups and also to their deities. The cord connects all three levels. To me this makes much sense and is a wonderful way to view the literal and the supernatural as all part of one eternal cord.

A prospective priestess might have a calling or become possessed by a deity. Such things are seen as normal and auspicious and invite possible initiation. Female initiates undergo many secret rites but some are known to the outside world. There is the tradition of making the initiate sit on four upturned cooking pots with their legs apart. It is seen as very bad should any of the pots break and the initiate wouldl be banished from that particular shrine as a result. The importance of the cooking pot is rated extremely highly. The pot is sometimes called 'fome' and represents the womb. Each shrine has a 'fome' and a stool. The stool is for a male deity to sit upon if it is invoked.

Although the men of the tribe control the blood ties of their family by keeping their sons within the family group and controlling the land of the tribe or family, it is the women who are the traders and entrepreneurs. This is reflected in their beliefs. A female initiate may also undergo scarification and the drinking of a sacrificed animal's blood. These traditions are seen as ways of strengthening the 'blood tie' to the deity who has called upon them. There are many traditional practices within Vodhun. Magic or 'witchcraft' that is both black and white is one such example. From healing to cursing, and all in between, some priestesses will be called upon to administer any one of these at any time. Rites of passage are regularly adhered to as are initiation rites, specific rituals and healing. Ancestral connections are also paid homage to but in a very specific and separate manner. The male ancestors are remembered by name and called upon as such whereas the female ancestors are all seen as one mother and can only be connected by the Vodhun or deity of each shrine. The doors of shrines are painted in colours that might resonate with today's Western witches. Each one has three colours, black, red and white. Red symbolises the contents of 'fome' or the womb of life and the 'hun' within, whereas black symbolises death. White symbolises the semen of the male. If the shrine has an upturned pot on its roof then it tells the other villagers that a vodhun or deity is present

This love of the crossroads of life extends to protective amulets, which represent protection from the crossing point of the void and all who pass through it. The cord of blood to the father is kept through the male lineage and the connection with the paternal land that the men are, like the trunk of the Hunde tree, rooted in. The women are seen as wild and not rooted until a man takes them as a wife. Women are viewed collectively as creatures akin to animals that have to be hunted down. This is not in any way deemed as derogatory, quite the opposite, the instinctive, intuitive fruit bearing woman is held in high regard. As a daughter she can marry and obtain a husband who will provide food and shelter for her and a safe place for her children. She must do most of the domestic chores but men also help out, depending on the time each person has available. She is responsible for the alchemy of cooking. Women earned the right to prepare the food because the 'fome' or pot is linked to the womb and the cooking process likened to gestation and birth. If a woman cannot cook it is seen as a bad omen. Such a woman might be infertile and unable to bear children, or she could be promiscuous and a threat to the stability of the marriages in the village. Perhaps most striking is the fact that the majority of spiritual elite in vodhun and voodoo are women!

All children 'belong' to their fathers; they can inherit land if there is any for descendants to inherit. This applies to male descendants in the first place and females secondly. A woman can sell spare produce, craft products, illegal alcohol, vodhun fetishes, pots, etc., and increase the family's wealth and status accordingly.

Each tribe will plant a 'Hunde Tree' in their village. This tree is sacred. It must be kept alive and its fruit left alone. The trunk of the tree represents the male energy and phallus and the fruit the female energy. To these people a tree can become a God and, therefore, must be treated with similar respect and reverence. The life force of the tree in this case is seen to be reflecting the health and virility of the tribe or village. One can see why the ancestors held this one in such high esteem. When split or cut it appears to bleed as it has a red resinous sap. It is also considered very bad luck to chop one down or cut it in any way.

The spiritual transcendence of the blood tie during rituals is often achieved by trance and dance and the setting up of a Vodhun shrine is no exception. During this ritual the whole village will attend and participate in the celebration of another deity acknowledging their tribe. Each priestess, or more rarely, priest, will pass their shrine down to the next initiate in line and is ultimately responsible for its upkeep and safety during its existence. The blood tie with the deity is strengthened with each ritual that involves any form of blood, be it from scarification, piercings, animal sacrifice or menstrual offerings. The blood tie with the land is created by the women through the men. By having their children in the village and being wives to men who live there they are creating the blood lines that might last for many generations. This might seem incredibly simplistic but their beliefs, rituals, traditional practices and relationships with each other and their deities are all integrated into their everyday life and this wholesome and holistic way of existing within their religion enables them to have secure identities and known roles. The mysterious side of their practices comes about through vodhun. Vodhun doesn't set out to deliberately control them but they are strongly affected by the magic vodhun exerts upon them. This God/Blood or divine blood mystery really gets to the roots of many belief systems that emerged from African traditions.

Haitian Voodoo

The many attempts by religious bodies and political powers to reduce the practice of Vodhun seems futile. This is a belief system so deeply entrenched in the very blood of its people, from conception to birth and on to death, that to eradicate it might be to deny the existence of the very people themselves.

Slavery has given African Traditional Paths global status. And although the people enslaved had no choice in their degradation and capture, they took their culture and belief systems with them. If one tiny bit of good came out of this horrendous time in mankind's history it was to open the world's eyes to the plethora of traditional paths that emerged from Africa. The slaves that found themselves in Haiti came predominantly from Benin, Angola and Nigeria. The people of Haiti were left alone, by and large, after being declared an independent republic and, apart from Catholicism being declared as the national religion by the departing French, it retained a connection with its roots.

The people of Haiti refer to their spirituality as 'serving the spirits'. These spirits can be live ones, dead ones and divine ones. All are inter-connected in the Haitian belief structure. Much like the Watchi, the Haitian peoples see all human and divine spirits as being interrelated. The health of the relationships between each type of spirit is the denominator of a person's state of well being at any one time. To the Haitians, healing comes top of their list of vodou practices to be carried out. This makes perfect sense. If you are taken from your home and placed on an island thousands of miles away to be enslaved by people whose language, culture and spiritual beliefs are all alien to you then turning to your own at times of ill health is natural. The priests and priestesses that were enslaved took their medicinal knowledge with them. They also took with them the wisdom of the spiritual world. The blood tie of each family would be known to the priests and the deities the families have rooted would also be known, but to practise what the Western world viewed as 'black magic' put their lives in even more danger than it already was. The one form of practice that might have been tolerated by the slave owners was herbal and spiritual medicine. Anything that saved them money and trouble and got a worker back on his or her feet must have been accepted by the greedy few who controlled them. But once slavery was abolished and the islanders were free to follow their own path again, it had already changed. The merging of the three dominant African traditions with Christianity created the creole style of vodou we are familiar with in places such as New Orleans. In Haiti the divine blood suffered greatly. Torn from their land and uprooted from the rest of their families, they sought to retain as much of their blood ties as possible. Only by family members sticking close together, and probable incest, could such blood lineages survive. The need to connect with the new land would also be strong as they wanted to root their deities to this place they found themselves in. But it wasn't easy. They were opposed by their slavemasters and suppressed by Catholicism.

Poverty and disease is rife in Haiti, even to this day. It is still an island republic where the elite few own most of the land and the wealth. The vast majority of Haitians are born into short life expectancy and suffering is the order of each day. To the believers in vodou, the spirits have much to do with this. The source belief that the cord of blood that ties them above and below to their kith and kin and to their ancestors, linked to their land and to the deities is, profound. Therefore, they adopt a pragmatic view. In their eyes they are born into this life because of their relationship with spirits. It is then their job to make the best of it. They don't have anything to aim for or much in the way of good education or future prospects, let alone any real advancement. Their blood tie to the family became stronger than the land tie for a while and this also shifted their beliefs. But they have vodou and the desire to heal one another and serve their spirits and that seems to keep them going.

One of the major changes that has taken place over successive generations is that the elder father or patriarch of the extended family is often called upon to double as the *oungan*, or 'priest', when that family serves the spirits. With their own hereditary priests and priestesses having been left behind, families had to improvise and the decision among the Haitian vodou practitioners was to elevate the elder male of any one family to the position of priest. This break from the traditional path of it being more of a feminine role to become a priestess was also a definitive change from previous vodhun traditions. The fome or blood tie of the family is still intact but the spiritual work is now carried out by virtue of patrimony and nothing else. The drastic increase in the numbers of family dying at an early age calls for family cemeteries and it is true to say that from slavery, the Caribbean voodoo and Haitian vodou almost shifted towards becoming more of a death cult than the previous tree of life cult on mainland Africa.

Hoodoo

Hoodoo is often confused with Voodoo but is quite distinctly different. Whereas Voodoo or Vodhun/Vodou is a religion, Hoodoo is more a mixture of various traditional magical practices. Hoodoo incorporates Jewish mysticism and borrows heavily from both the Kabbalah and the Old Testament, often mixed in with Native American spells, African traditional folk magic and Christian mysticism. It is a potent blend indeed, and one that might, at first glance, seem unlikely to work. However, it does, and those who practise hoodoo certainly believe in it. Hoodoo has made its way into a lot of blues music and is often found in places such as New Orleans alongside Creole Voodoo. It is mostly practised on the US mainland.

Blood Mysteries

The Bible features a lot in Hoodoo. It is used as a protective amulet, as a source of magical spells and Hoodoo practitioners see the underlying magic or mysticism woven deeply throughout its pages. Psalms are often used for spell work and are repeated three times to make them work. Two Psalms often used in Hoodoo are number 37 for protection and number 91 for removing jinxes or hexes. One example is using the 91st Psalm for Uncrossing or Jinx removing purposes. These words are seen as magical in their own right. Chanting is not found in Hoodoo. Hoodoo practitioners believe in an ultimate creator God and identify him with the God of the Old Testament or Jewish Bible. They view him as the archmagician and the one who is both creator and healer rolled into one. As many Hoodoo practitioners are raised on Catholicism and Santeria it is not that surprising to find these beliefs in their conjuring. Indeed, the very word Hoodoo is meant to mean conjure or potion; it is the magical act of changing and influencing events.

Some conjuring requires blood, either blood of sacrificed animals or menstrual blood, depending on the spell being cast. It is important to note that animal sacrifice is rare in Hoodoo and more often found in Voodoo, Vodhun, Palo and other paths. This most probably stems from the African element as it is frequently found in West Coast African traditional Vodhun, as mentioned earlier. Sometimes parts of animals are used as the energy, or life force, of the creature sacrificed that is imbued into one part of the dead animal. This also reminds us of the muti practice in Africa. The belief that the life force of a person or animal can be carried in the blood is definitely found here and using this energy for conjuring is considered to be one of the most powerful spells one can cast.

Often any Hoodoo involving animal sacrifice or blood being spilt is seen as 'black magic' and is attributed to Satanic practises. This is rarely ever the case. The magic is only ever as good or bad as the intention behind it. Some Hoodoo practitioners, much like any other sort of witch, will deliberately use their abilities and knowledge to perform 'black' or deliberately destructive magic, but it is almost impossible to estimate how many do. Those who work 'black magic' rarely shout about it. Animal sacrifice does still occur in some traditions, but it is not as common as it used to be. This sort of Hoodoo is falling out of fashion and generally frowned upon. The traditional Voodoo doll is probably more to do with root work conjuring or Hoodoo than Voodoo, with the smearing of blood upon it or inside it being a popular thing to do to add magical weight and energetic strength to the Hoodoo one is trying to achieve.

People who use Hoodoo aren't always massively religious despite using the Bible so much in their conjuring. They do see certain characters in the Bible as being magicians or conjurors with Moses, Elijah and Christ being highly regarded. A European grimoire, The Sixth and Seventh Book of Moses — a system that borrows from the Jewish Kabbalah — is used a lot by Hoodoo practitioners. Another which they like to draw from is John George Holman's 'Pow-wows or Long Lost Friend'. These essentially Western European magical books are used for guidance and instruction in Hoodoo conjuring. The belief that a book in itself is powerful, whether one has actually read it or not, is upheld by Hoodoo practitioners. So they often choose to carry a Bible on them at all times for protection.

Most Hoodoo is used for healing, protection, divining, results magic and spell casting. Blood does come into it, but not as much as it used to. Menstrual blood is seen as the most mystical and powerful of all. This, as we have discovered, is commonly believed in by all traditions that utilise it. It is also important to realise that not all sacrificial magic is negative or black magic. Though it might seem extreme to us sometimes, the killing of an animal can be used to work very powerful healing magic, or magic to bring loved ones back, or to heal wounds between peoples — the list is endless. Many Hoodoo practitioners are also necromancers and both ancestral work and contact with the deceased is common. They believe it is easier for the dead to carry out magical work on our behalf as they are closer to us than other more divine manifestations or spirits or lwa. Offering your own blood during a Hoodoo working is fairly common, and a Hoodoo practitioner will often bring blood into his or her conjuring.

Quimbanda

Many variants, or remnants, of African Traditional Religions made their way to central and south America during the slave exportations. One such example that practices occasional blood rituals and sacrifices is Quimbanda. Once known as a type of Macumba that split into two branches, Quimbanda and Umbanda, it has kept the African black magic label. And unlike Umbanda it doesn't have strong Catholic content. The three main types of spirit in quimbanda are Ogum, Exus and Pomba Giras. Ogum is a creator and war spirit and also linked with metallurgy who seems rarely called upon. Exus are male and often seen as devilish, mercurial and immoral. And Pomba Giras are female spirits that are all various aspects and faces of femininity, often seen as fiery, passionate and sulphurous in their natures. Both seem to represent extremes. Exu is Pomba Gira's consort.

The tradition has a long history of initiation and during one initiate to a Pomba Gira (there are many and the initiate is identified prior to initiation), ceremonial cuts are made in the skin into which specific herbs are pressed home. This powerful process of blending the initiates blood with the spiritual presence of Pomba Gira, or Exu depending on the initiation, deepens the bond between the living and the spirit. It serves to identify you to Pomba Gira or Exu.

Both Pomba Giras and Exus are guardians of the many crossroads a person will encounter in life. Because of this, rituals often include the necessity to visit a T-shaped crossroads or, in the case of Pomba Giras and Exus, at regular crossroads. They are both known as beings connected with marginal spaces and crossroads. It seems that when called upon they offer up choices and options waiting for the initiate to use his or her spiritual knowledge and good judgement before making the decision on which road to take. Liminal spaces such as beaches, in the case of some Pomba Giras, are opportune places to listen more carefully to spirits, as important messages are often relayed here and offerings into the sea can be made.

Quimbanda is a magical tradition with precise formulas and instructions on how to conduct rituals, each of which has a specific purpose. The intent must be followed through with the relevant ritual and the results must be accepted as that which is right for you. With this in mind it is important to understand that both the male and female forces of Quimbanda will know you, truly know you, no corner of your psyche will be kept secret from them. Total honesty is the only way forward. I have also encountered this with Germanic and Norse and Egyptian deities. They are not straightforward — they test people, often to the limits of their inner strength and abilities. Some doors they open at the crossroads will be traps for you to fall in, or lessons you don't really need to learn, but presented in an alternative manner so as to disguise their true purpose. Many of the rituals are difficult to undertake as they involve procuring items that might not always be easy to obtain. Many include the need for living animal sacrifice, an example of which is the black cockerel. This is sometimes offered up to an Exu during a ritual where one hopes to harm another. This aspect of Quimbanda is partly why it is seen as 'Black Magic'. I once wrote in a book on West Country Witchcraft that magic has no colour because it is all colours and it is the desired result that defines the positive or negative outcome. If we take the matter of say, revenge into our own hands, are we not merely acting out the balance? Or what some see as karma? Does it matter if we take the opportunity sometimes to do this ourselves rather than wait for the universe to kick back? Naturally not all petitions of this nature to an Exu are for vengeance.

Animals that are often chosen for sacrifice include pigeons, cockerels, goats, sheep and toads. Sometimes the sacrifice is bound and the moment of death and offering is at the end of the ritual. Occasionally the blood drawn from the sacrifice is poured into a communal bowl and passed around the congregation and taken by each member. Quimbanda is not alone in still making these offerings to spirits.

Quimbanda seems a vibrant visceral tradition that is definitely not for the fainthearted. Those I know of on this path, and they are only a handful, seem strong intelligent people well versed in life and embrace it with full vigour! They are also very magical and always get results!

Religious Blood Rituals

A Ritual associated with Blood Sacrifices

I don't choose to offer up the life of an animal in ritual even though some of the spirits I connect with might ask it of others. I am always happy to give of my own blood but accept that if a greater sacrifice needs making, a price might need paying in other ways.

I work with Azaz-el whose complex mythology would fill another book. Before anyone gets confused thinking he is merely a fallen angel or demon, I thought I'd point this out. I see him as an ancient shaman whose tribe were goat herders and this is the aspect of him I connect with. So for the sake of this book it is his goat deity aspect I wish to draw from and make contact with. As the formative scapegoat, his existence in the Hebrew mindset was very real and one that they felt all their sins should be cast out and upon. Considering how many poor goats met their end this way I feel drawn to pay homage to him. It is ironic that the live offering is the one we honour here rather than the burnt or dead one. But since the majority of the poor goats sent out into the wilderness had their legs broken or worse to prevent them returning, they died a terrible protracted death to wash the sins of the Hebrew peoples away.

Azaz-el Calling

Altar: Red cloth — 5 candles red and/or black — a metal chalice filled with red wine or red liquor/spirit (he also likes a strong honey rum). A metal senser.

A goat skull with horns (Painting his sigil on it helps)
Inverted pentagram optional
A live and dried dead red rose head.

A large stone painted black with his sigil in red and a chain that you can break easily with a small hammer

Food and drink offerings — goats eat pretty much everything, except meat.

Preparatory bath, and if you are female he always appreciates you using cosmetics, especially eye makeup. Robe and/or clothing according to personal preference; he also likes skyclad.

Sterile blade or needles.

Best times are dark moon, solar eclipses, full moon.

Time – midnight.

Face east if possible.

Open yourself up and raise energy.

Calling

Begin your ritual in darkness.

Spend a few minutes imagining Azaz-el and everything you have found out about him before lighting your candles.

I call upon Azaz-el, he of the black sun whose birth caused it to burn more strongly.

I call upon the son of Samael and Lilith whose home is the dry mountainous deserts.

I call upon he of the wilderness whose name is Azaz-el.

I call upon he who is strongest of divinity and cannot be broken

I call upon he who dwells in Duedal and is released once more

I call upon he who seeks to liberate us from binds and chains and aids us to find our own inherent divine power

I call upon the blighted, the cursed, the unclean bird!

Hail Azaz-el messenger of the Gods

Hail Azaz-el the scapegoat

Hail Azaz-el the Horned God of the people

Hail Azaz-el the fallen one

Hail Azaz-el the alchemist of souls

Hail Azaz-el angel of metals and antinomy

Hail Azaz-el the bound in the fiery pit

(Take up your hammer and smash the chain saying…)

Once, twice, thrice I strike at the chains that bind you so you

may fly free with wings that black out the sun once more!!
(Top up incense)
Hail to thee who is most feared and revered Lord of the Earth
Sovereign of humanity
Eternal flame of Lilith, she who screeches as dusk falls and is Queen of the Night
Protect me from your black light that it may enlighten and not singe
(pause and increase energy- use whatever method you have been taught)
I call he who picks his way carefully among the flock
And he who is the true shepherd of the cloven hooved
Whose flesh, skin, blood and bones have been sacrificed to us
And to whom a live goat is sent out to on the day of atonement of sins that
Only Azaz-el can cleanse us of
Purge us to our cores that we may tremble in your presence
Hail Melek Taus the Peacock Angel whose likeness is cast upon thee
Hail son of Samael whose title The Satan has been cast upon he
Hail son of Lilith whose title Queen of Demons has been cast upon she
Hail brother of Lucifer whose title The Devil is cast upon he
Accept these offerings of food and drink and incense and blood set here in your honour
Come to me/us this dark moon night
(Make offerings)
Hear our pleas....
Fill me/us with your strength
Protect me/us from harm
Guide me/us in your wisdom
Help us pick our way through the world carefully mindful of the steps we take and how sure footed we must be

Aid me/us to be free of the tyranny and false laws placed upon me/us

Enhance our lives with loves and lusts and passions beyond measure

Let us revel in all forms of ecstasy free of prejudice and limitation if it be our will to do so

Liberate us from closed thinking and open our minds to seeing more clearly the journey we take in our lives

Grant us peace of mind and heart that if we love well and live well we will be well

Allow us the freedom to take responsibility for our actions and accept the consequences

And know that it is our mortal role to learn from our mistakes

Accept here these drops of my life force I give to tie my soul to yours and accept me as your initiated child a true willing sacrifice given freely in your name.

(Let five drops of blood fall on the incense)

Sit in quiet meditation and enjoy your unique communion with this ancient goat deity.

And, when ready, give thanks and close.

The above is a straightforward calling that could, if someone wished it, be adapted for any particular desired result. It would be possible to add a different intent to it other than the enlightening petition included.

CHAPTER 7
Cannibalism

Tribes in Papua New Guinea were made famous for their cannibalism as recently as the 1970s. A rare form of mad cow disease similar to CJD seemed to plague a tribe that practiced endocannibalism. This ancient practice of eating deceased relatives occurs all over the world in primal cultures. Evidence of the disease was found in highest levels in brain and spinal tissue. Although the tribe also practised exocannibalism, the practice of eating enemies, through warfare and targeted murders, it was the endocannibalism that got them into the severest trouble. It was their practice of consuming the brain of the deceased person that meant the women were passing the infection on at the genetic level to future generations. When researched by scientists such as Carleton Gajdusek and Baruch Blumberg, the tribe was open about their enjoyment of the taste of human flesh and saw no problem with it at all. Once the tribe was enlightened as to the risks they were exposed to this form of cannibalism reduced in popularity. And 'Kuru,' as they named the mystery illness, also decreased with it.

During the Second World War it was common for tribes

in Papua New Guinea to eat Japanese prisoners of war. To a cannibalistic tribe this not only meant extra free meat but was also a way of absorbing the bravery of their enemy whilst eradicating the need to feed a captured soldier. Taken at its simplest form this makes perfect common sense and one can understand why cannibalism worked as a very effective deterrent. Can we really imagine how terrified you would be to be caught by cannibals? Being held a captive of war and tortured and or starved would be bad enough, but knowing they might eat you could invoke a far greater terror.

Cannibalism could be seen as the ultimate taboo, but it hasn't always been viewed this way and many of our own ancient ancestors might well have partaken of the odd human morsel or two. It is to Christopher Columbus that we have to look for the origin or etymology of the word. He happened upon a tribe called Carib — the word we now associate with the Caribbean. These tribes were alleged to have practised cannibalism. His people mispronounced Carib and managed to make it sound like Canib, giving rise to the word 'cannibal' that we are familiar with today.

Reasons for cannibalism are many and varied and evidence of it occurs all over the world, from ancient times right up until the present day. Spiritual cannibalism such as exocannibalism, when one tribe deliberately seeks to consume the human flesh of another tribe, is rife where aggressive warrior tribes co-exist too close to each other and are fighting over resources and land. Conversely, consuming the flesh of ones own tribe is described as endocannibalism and is more to do with wishing to honour one's loved ones who have just passed on in the ultimate way. This sort of compassionate absorption of a tribal member makes sure that the spirit of the deceased lives on through the entire tribe. Amazonian Wari practised this and it might well be the origins of all subsequent forms of cannibalism. While we might find the thought of laying granny out in state and carving pieces off her corpse to share around the family disgusting and abhorrent, we have to remember that our own roots may well stem from such actions. Often what we find distasteful today was greatly respected and honorable in the past. With our modern day values and ethics we shy from such activity, and science has taught us that eating corpses isn't always the healthy option. Yet our ancestors knew no different.

What seems to have stopped this sort of activity in most cultures is the rise of organised book religions with very specific rules and regulations concerning all eating habits and rituals. In the majority of modern traditions, rituals for the treatment of the deceased moved right away from any form of cannibalistic format, seeing the corpse as unclean. As the rise of Abrahamic paths grew and exploded all over the globe, so previous cultures took on board the new ethics and morals associated with whichever path they chose, Judaism, Christianity and Islam being the main three although Buddhism and Hinduism are also non-cannibalistic paths. All appear to have roughly the same view on the hygiene aspects of handling dead bodies. It would seem that at some point mankind began to make a correlation between sickness and touching cadavers. This is possible, but it very much depends on how the person died, and of what. Any virulent or bacterial infection can still be transmitted after death, and hotter countries have greater risks of bodies going sour more quickly than cooler ones. It seems as though common sense and priestly decisions regarding the afterlife also permeated these affected societies. What we now consider to be more civilized behaviors have their roots in changing beliefs and religious and political infrastructures. These changes might well have been introduced slowly and gradually to move people away from risks associated with eating human flesh. Looked at dispassionately there is no difference between a dead human body and a dead animal body. Both die and decompose — it is as simple as that. One is treated in a ritual manner to allow for human consumption and the other is tucked away in a hole in the ground, tomb or is cremated. But we don't eat diseased animals. And this is probably the crux of the matter as neither should we eat a diseased person. Most people die of wear and tear, heart disease, cancers, strokes, pneumonia, etc., but some die of highly infectious and easily transmitted infections; some, like the tribes in Papua New Guinea discovered, pass these on genetically by eating the diseased person's flesh. New awareness of health risks do play a large part in the shift from one way of dealing with death to another, and it also seems highly likely that in an area where diseases such as these were rife, so cannibalism would fall from favour. In areas with less negative associations however, cannibalism still thrived. Fear of disease does seem to have been the largest factor in reducing occurrences of cannibalism in modern times but it does, in lesser degrees, still happen to this day.

There is certainly archaeological evidence for it among most ancient tribes all over the globe, from Australia and New Zealand to Europe and pretty much everywhere in between. When archaeologists look for evidence of cannibalism, among bones they have several markers to go by. Panche Hadzi-Andonov in his book Cannibalism and Archaeology cites skull invasion and crushing open, burnt bones, missing vertebra, dismemberment and bone breakage as some of the clues they look for. There have been excavations of Neanderthal bones in Croatia displaying many of these signs, including cut marks on bones which indicate that the flesh was removed after death.

The reasons for, and purpose of cannibalism vary. Some are most definitely religious and follow beliefs that in absorbing the flesh of a deceased relative one can take on the literal energy of that person, as we have already touched upon. Famine is another contender and is ery likely as the human race has had to survive through many of these over its history. Even in Egypt there is evidence that in 1201 BCE, from wall art of the time, people were driven to cannibalism.

War is yet another reason for cannibalism, as consuming the flesh of your enemy is believed in some ancient traditions to give you some of his, or her, strength. Often this stemmed from the respect one had for one's enemies. For example, if you deemed the enemy tribe as particularly fierce and fearless then these are qualities which consuming the dead might transfer. This bloody transference is so incredibly basic a premise it is not at all surprising it is found among tribal cultures all over the world. We often hear of Native American tribes eating the still-beating hearts of their enemies — this being where a person's bravery is often thought to stem from. Scalping, another bloody tradition, also provokes great fear and means a trophy of each battle is acquired. Much exocannibalism is trophy based and often lacks ritual, as it is taken during the fighting, but endocannibalism is more sedate.

Reverence and ceremony abide in these rituals. Bodies are washed and prepared in traditional manners by priests or shamans or witchdoctors. All of a tribe would be expected to attend and partake. Each tribe might deal differently with the remains after consumption, but special ritual knives would be used that have been specially made for this purpose and never used for anything else. Each tribe would have their own way of sectioning and selecting portions for consumption, with muscle flesh being the most popular. Offal is also eaten sometimes as are brains. Importance would be given to varying parts of the body. Some tribes held the heart in highest esteem, some brain, some muscle but each has their own peculiarities. And some would drain the blood for drinking whereas some would drain it and dispose of it, not seeing it as important at all.

Modern Cannibalism

In the vast majority of today's societies cannibalism is not illegal, and this came as quite a surprise to me when I found out. It is deemed as socially unacceptable, but not always seen as a crime, depending on circumstances. It seems to depend on the situation that gives rise to the cannibalistic act. If the person is murdered or grievously injured to attain edible human flesh then these crimes are charged as such, but not the actual act of consumption.

A famous example of a modern day crime involving cannibalism is that of Nicolas Claux in 1994. He was convicted of the murder of a 34-year-old man but this wasn't the story that shocked the world. It was news that whilst he had been working at a children's hospital he had been taking the flesh of dead children's bodies home to eat. He admitted to eating it and said he preferred it raw to steak. He was also believed to be a Satanist. Satan gets blamed with a few such crimes, from time to time, such as the French case of Japanese student Issei Sagawa. He failed to win the favors of a particular lady so shot her and posthumously sexually assaulted her, and then ate her breasts and buttocks. Although he was incarcerated for a while in a French institution for the mentally impaired, he later returned to Japan where, after a relatively short period of prison, he was set free and has been ever since. Most weird of all is that he has profited from his crime and managed to attain celebrity status. Another case that has links with old horny is that of Dmitry Dyomin and two other cohorts who abducted a fifteen year old girl in Kiev. She was murdered and Dmitry is said to have eaten her tongue. He was also said to be a fan of Satanism. This form of epicurean cannibalism is the rarest. People who eat human flesh, merely because some higher power has allegedly endorsed it or encouraged it, or purely for the nutritional or taste value don't often occur these days.

But criminal cannibalism does hit the news occasionally and shock us all when it does. And with stories such as Thomas Harris's Silence of the Lambs from the Hannibal trilogy becoming blockbuster films, our fascination with this darkest of criminally related activity pervades.

The inspiration for both the character of Buffalo Bill in Silence of the Lambs and Norman Bates from Hitchcock's film Psycho came from a character caught in Plainfield Wisconsin, named Eddie Gein. This loner was arrested as a suspect in a robbery but what detectives found at his house still haunts those involved in the case today. The house was described as filthy and stinking of putrid flesh. A decapitated corpse hung from a beam and many seemingly ordinary household objects such as lamp shades were made of human skin. Eddie Gein preyed on women and made himself transvestite skin suits from his victims and also claimed to eat their flesh. It is unlikely that Satan was in any way involved in this crime as it was more likely to have stemmed from Eddie's overbearing and strict religious Christian upbringing. His mother had a negative view of sex that for some reason she linked with her relationship with God and encouraged her boys away from it. It is possible that being married to a weak alcoholic had something to do with this, but it was an extreme and antisocial reaction nonetheless. They were told how angry and upset God would be if he knew about their 'dirty' thoughts. Sex was reduced to an unpleasant and unfortunate yet necessary action for the production of children and nothing else. Her constant verbal abuse kept them on her straight and narrow path.

Eddie respected his mother by all accounts and even tried hard to live up to her impossible standards. The boys were discouraged from having friends but Eddie did do well at school. This kind of unloving, psychotic and overprotective environment can sometimes give rise to even worse behaviour in those raised by such people. His father was an alcoholic, so he was definitely dredging deep emotional depths and yet came across as weak. He doted on his mother seeing her as the epitome of goodness and was devastated when she died of a series of strokes. His adoration and almost Goddess worship of her was to manifest in one of the most bizarre and extraordinary crimes ever. It seems as though his lust for mother went beyond the skin in the most literal sense. His desire for her transmuted into acts of murder and cannibalism giving rise to the thought that he loved her so much that he couldn't be consumed by her, so he consumed others in her place. A disturbing tale.

A cannibalistic story quite unlike any other that could be construed as epicurean cannibalism is that of Armin Meiwes in 2001. The world was shocked to hear that he had placed an advertisement on the internet asking for someone to offer themselves up to become his dinner. This very peculiar and deranged man from Roteburg in Germany wanted a 'well built 18-30 year old to be slaughtered and then consumed'. Amazingly someone actually answered this and the two men are said to have first met on Christmas day. In March, Bernd Jurgen Brandes arrived at Armin's home to offer himself up for dinner. It is believed there were strong sexual overtones and desires behind both men's motives for doing this. Brandes wished Armin to bite his penis off, which failed so it was severed by a knife. Brandes wanted both men to eat his penis. This wasn't overly successful either and even after frying it they found the dismembered member 'too chewy' as Brandes describes on the tape. The penis was then fed to Armins dog. Armin then left Brandes to bleed almost to the point of death in his bath after plying him with pain killers and alcohol whilst he coolly sat down to read a book.

Once ready, Armin removed Brandes to his pre-prepared slaughter room. He proceeded to kiss him and then he stabbed him in the throat and killed him. He hung the body up on a meat hook and carved the flesh off the bones most of which was then frozen and consumed by Armin over the next ten months. He placed his original advertisement in Cannibal Café, a website dedicated to the subject matter. The story defied credibility and yet the unfortunate court room had to sit through this and both watch and hear the act being performed by Armin Meiwes. His initial sentence of eight years for manslaughter was eventually overturned at a re-trial where he was found guilty of murder and, somewhat less surprisingly, he is now serving a life sentence for murder. Sexual epicurean cannibalism might not appear to stem from any particular bloodlust but one wonders if at a subconscious level it is? What is it about this form of cannibalism that drives people to commit crimes such as this?

Another famous example of this variety of sexual/epicurean cannibalism is that of Jeffrey Dahmer from Wisconsin. He lured young men to his apartment where he would sedate them and then murder and dismember them. It is said that he both consumed and experimented with their remains — there are horrific tales of injecting hydrochloric acid into their brains to turn them into compliant sexual zombies. He was also into necrophilia and liked to indulge in sexual acts with the corpses. He was an alcoholic and was turfed out of the army for this. His early crimes took place whilst he was living at his grandmother's house but once he lived on his own, the pace picked up considerably. His main motivation seems sexual and aimed towards much younger men and boys making him also a paedophile. Whether this all stemmed from severe repressed homosexuality issues or whether he himself was abused is not conclusively known. He was eventually caught and charged with no less than 17 murders and sent to prison to serve multiple life sentences. However, an inmate took matters into his own hands and he was beaten to death on 28th November in 1994. These kinds of sexually motivated forms of cannibalism are very rare but others include Andrei Chikatilo, a Ukrainian serial killer who raped, killed and ate up to 50 victims before finally being charged and executed in Rostov in 1994. And Albert Fish from New York who kidnapped, raped and murdered a ten-year-old girl before eating part of her remains and sending a letter describing his acts in detail to her family. He was also caught and executed.

Whether any form of bloodlust also fuels these criminals on in their quests for deviant illegal sexual gratification is unclear but possible. Bloodlust is very potent and could, in theory, increase the desire for committing further revolting acts without these criminals even being aware of it. It is hard for most civilized .peaceful people to imagine anyone wanting to perform such acts, let alone try and understand them, but the primal beast is under the surface of every man and woman in the world. Although very few of us are sexually deviant to such degrees, the animal within will out, under the right circumstances.

This takes us on to the last type for which we have modern-day examples — of necessity or famine-induced cannibalism. The evidence for this variety of can be found all over the world. Only sheer desperation will drive some people to eat the flesh of another human being, and this is in some respects understandable. Although very few of us will ever go to these lengths it has occurred as recently in our history as the 1970s. A rugby team from Uruguay were flying out to Chile to play in a match when their plane crashed in bad weather high up in the Chilean mountains. 16 members of the 45 aboard managed to survive against all odds for over two months in the freezing mountainous conditions. They did this by living off of the remains of the dead passengers. A film, Alive, was made of their story which touched the hearts of those who heard it, but also provoked many ethical and moral discussions and debates. Many people found themselves asking the same question, 'would I also do this if it were my only way to survive?'. They were eventually rescued and no one was charged with any criminal acts because none had actually been carried out. The people who died were accidently killed by the crash and therefore already dead. This is probably the most benign form of cannibalism.

Unsurprisingly I have avoided giving any form of ritual where cannibalism is concerned.

Chapter 8
Medical

Once you delve into the medical world, blood seems to be everywhere you look. And this is not at all surprising. It is to Egypt we travel first for they were pioneers in the world of surgery.

These ancient surgeons were active as long ago as 3000BCE with Imhotep being the first recorded to practice anything like what we would now consider medicine. The belief that demons and evil spirits were the cause of most problems was prevalent, and spells and incantations abound on papyrus, yet this went hand in hand with quite sophisticated abilities for their time. They were adept at setting simple fractures, rudimentary dentistry, and circumcision (they are believed to be the originators of this practice) among other things, and evidence also points to them being the first who ever practised any form of cosmetic surgery.

All those from other countries who visited ancient Egypt were amazed at their prowess. They even managed to create false eyes and other forms of prosthetics, thus proving that limb amputation also took place. Pliny the Elder mentioned them as did Herodotus, the Greek historian, in 440 BCE who recorded their medical practices as did Hippocrates, who is considered to be the father of classical medicine. It is not surprising that the ancient Egyptians became such early medical and surgical people. Their mummification process meant that those involved in it became proficient and knowledgeable of basic anatomy and physiology. They understood the connection with the blood carrying nutrition and waste, and pulses were roughly understood as being connected. These presumptions were uncannily accurate. Their view of the heart and brain however were not and ancient Egyptians swapped roles for these two organs. But they did have the very simple idea that just as blood flowed through veins and arteries, so air and other energetic substances also flowed through us.

Blood had importance to ancient Egyptians, and was even consumed as a life enhancing and beneficial force. Some coffins were found with spells concerning the belief that devouring hearts and drinking blood is good for health and will aid someone in their afterlife towards immortality. Spells with words such as: *'You devoured their hearts, so that you might live; you drank their blood, so that you might live'* are commonplace.

Probably the most famous case of 'Vampirism' in Ancient Egypt surrounds Sekhmet, the goddess of healing and pestilence. In a story known as *The Destruction of Mankind*, the human race plots against the sun god, Ra. In retaliation, Ra sends the goddess Hathor to lay waste to humanity. The instant that the blood touches her lips, Hathor is transformed into the bloodthirsty and aggressive Sekhmet, who slaughters so many that she wades in their blood up to her knees. This spell is similar to descriptions of predatory animals who live in the Egyptian desert, who 'eat hearts and drink blood'. This also links in with the story of Sekhmet who, with her leonine head, takes on the attributes of the predator.

Shezmu is a fascinating character. In addition to being the Head Chef of the dead king, Shezmu is also responsible for certain punishments for those who do not live their lives in accordance with Egyptian morality. His job is to place bodies in his wine press in order to squeeze their blood from them, in which he then forces them to swim. Shezmu has sometimes been depicted with a leonine head, again emphasising the attributes of the predator that link in with the popular story of Sekhmet.

In all these instances, blood represents two things — life and power. The actions of the Egyptian 'Vampires' were a form of dominance over others. To consume the blood of another was to increase your own power, whilst at the same time robbing them of theirs. Egyptian Vampires did not battle with their curse in an attempt to regain their soul. They did not seduce their prey in order to feed. They most certainly did not sparkle. If Ancient Egypt is anything to go by, Vampires are meant to be predators, pure and simple.

Most of us have heard of bloodletting, that ancient practice of deliberately allowing blood to flow from a sick person in order to release the illness. This stems from the belief that evil demons or spirits were responsible for many diseases and sicknesses. And in the age prior to knowledge of germs and viruses our ancestors had to explain illness somehow and chose to place the blame on external and infernal beings bent on causing suffering. When we think of this practice, leeches come to mind. The use of leeches to encourage deliberate bleeding goes back many thousands of years. Leeches have been used by many countries and were mentioned in the ancient Indian Ayurvedic Texts. A leech is basically a type of segmented worm that mostly lives in fresh water. Hippocrates, the founder of Greek medicine, believed there were four main important bodily fluids that had to be in balance in order for a person to be healthy. And these were:

Choleric: Yellow bile, related to the Gall Bladder and to the element of fire which, it was believed would lead to bad temper and anger, if in excess.

Melancholic: Black bile, associated with the spleen and the element of earth. Would lead to insomnia and irritation if there was too much.

Phlegmatic: Phlegm, associated with the brain and the element of water. They believed it was responsible for rationality, and too much might lessen emotions

Sanguine: The blood, related to the liver and the element of air. They believed this dictated how brave and optimistic a person was.

These so called 'humors' were the basis for much diagnosing. Blood isn't one of the humors but we still use some of the terms today. Colic comes from the term Choleric, and Cholera also finds its etymology here.

The first to correctly identify the circulation was an Arab physician, Ibn al-Nafis, in 1242. He was the first person to give descriptions of both the coronary and pulmonary circulatory systems. His work also refuted the previous Greek 'humors' as he went on to identify various body systems and organs, along with their purpose.

The Romans did well by becoming aware that good hygiene played a large part in avoiding sickness and ill health and they were also very adept surgeons. This hygiene knowledge took British people much longer to re-learn after Roman occupation and even the black plague didn't stop us throwing our faeces into the street. Not until the Victorians built the great sewers did we begin to improve our sanitary standards. And we also owe the Victorians much for the advancements in medicine and knowledge concerning the medical uses of blood.

The history of blood transfusions begins in 1628 with William Harvey, the first to demonstrate how the blood circulated around the body 400 years after Ibn al-Nafis. He was succeeded by Sir Christopher Wren in 1657 who used Harveys equipment to demonstrate how fluids could be injected into animals. The first

Medical

ever successful transfusion on an animal was carried out in 1666 by Richard Lower. And a year later in 1667, the diarist Samuel Pepys recorded the experiment that took place of transfusing blood from one dog to another. There was then a long gap in the history of this discovery and it wasn't until 1818 that Dr James Blundell conducted successful transfusions on women suffering post partum bleeding (haemorrhaging after childbirth).

By 1900 a Dr Karl Landsteiner from Vienna made a landmark discovery which helped to explain why so many attempts at transfusion proved unsuccessful. He found that there were 4 basic blood groups in human beings and that we all fall into one of them. The blood groups of A, B, AB and O were born. He found the solution to over 270 years worth of experimenting.

By the Great War of 1914-1918 it had been found that blood has a much longer shelf life if chilled and that if you add sodium citrate to it you can slow down the rate that it clots. The British Red Cross were the first to launch a blood donating service and began by asking their own members to give blood. In 1931 the first UK blood banks service was set up in Ipswich. By the outbreak of the Second World War in 1939 there were four blood banks up and running in major cities in the UK, and a year later regional blood donations centres were opened all over the country.

After the the end of the war, in 1946 The National Blood Service was set up and launched along with the NHS. It wasn't until 1975 that glass bottles were replaced by plastic bags to contain, store and use the donated blood. The discovery of HIV and AIDS in the eighties meant that screening for it became necessary and it was introduced in 1986, followed by screening for Hepatitis C in 1991. The most recent advancement in the transfusion service was in 1999 with the introduction of Nucleic Acid & Amplification Technology coming into use to detect even the earliest signs of any viruses in the donated blood, making the transfusion service even safer.

Bloodletting

There is little or no evidence to verify whetherusing leeches to encourage bleeding actually cured anyone of any particular illness or disease; many recovered on their own through their own immune systems fighting off whatever had infected them, but the belief in the power of bloodletting was huge.

Strangely enough, leeches have found their way back into modern medicine. From the 1980s onwards they have been used for people who are intolerant of anti-coagulant drugs. In certain types of cosmetic surgical procedures where is it imperative for blood to keep flowing through veins close to the skin as part of the healing process, leeches are used. By applying a leech to the flap of skin that you need a good blood supply fed to, it is possible to prevent congestion

Sometimes bloodletting was more aggressive than merely allowing a leech to have some supper. Occasionally incisions were made and larger amounts of blood let. This was usually in the case of suspected demonic possession, where the demon would be ordered out of the person's body via the let blood. This form of bloodletting was fraught with danger. Sometimes too much blood was let this way and patients died as a result of the attempted healing. Other times secondary infections occurred as a result of not using a sterile blade.

It is possible that letting up to a pint of blood did make people feel a bit better. If you get rid of a percentage of the fluid that the infection is being carried in then you would feel lightened by its loss. And, if you were healthy enough to replace it with new blood of your own, it is possible your body would also replace it with the required amount of fresh new anti-bodies to fight the infection. With milder bacterial and viral problems, this might have helped slightly. But in most cases one presumes it was not beneficial to recovery and only served to further weaken the patient.

Medical

Jehovah's Witnesses and blood transfusions

The majority of Jehovahs Witnesses adhere to a 1945 doctrine that forbids them from either giving or receiving whole or even part blood products. By following texts in the Old Testament in Genesis, Leviticus and Acts they believe it is against the law of their God to indulge in any blood products. Their food must also be blood free. The rules are that the transfusion of allogeneic whole blood, or of its constituents of red cells, white cells, platelets or plasma is expressly forbidden as are transfusions of pre-operative self-donated autologous blood. They do allow blood to be taken and returned to a patient, as in dialysis for example and, they have a long list other blood related medical practices that they do permit. They also allow fractions of blood material to be transfused but are quite specific in which fractions can be permitted. If any of their members breaks this law and allow whole blood products to be transfused then they are shunned by the Witnesses.

In many cases, doctors are able to offer a wider variety of blood fractions for transfusions as the science of breaking the blood down into its component parts and offering bloodless surgery has advanced considerably since the discovery of HIV and AIDS. This doesn't help the JW members who have already died through refusing transfusions however.

To many people their literal take on these spiritual laws seems ridiculous and in many ways it is. The advice or doctrine was included in these texts as good advice to people living in a time prior to refrigeration whose hygiene was not as good as we have today. Modern life and science has informed us that it is not required to be so stringent. We can now prepare and store food more easily and safely and blood is thoroughly tested before being given to people, so risks to life are far lower. This might have been good, common-sense advice back then, but really doesn't apply to those on an Abrahamic path today, hence most modern day Christians, Jews and Muslims are quite happy to both give and accept blood donations. Thankfully in many countries the religious wishes of the parents of Jehovah's Witnesses are now often overturned if the child is under 15. Once over this age this can still be the case, unless the young person themselves objects to a transfusion. Their views and practices regarding blood transfusions are constantly being argued about throughout the society of Witnesses themselves and by the medical profession. It would be nice to think that one day common sense will prevail and that the society will allow their members the freedom of choice in a non-discriminating way.

Heart Surgery

Most surgical operations will involve having to deal with blood. Even a small cut or graze to the skin produces the red stuff. And thanks to coagulants, unless you sever a vein or artery, the bleeding usually stops very quickly without much intervention. But heart surgery is where the real complication of dealing with blood begins. The heart has four chambers, two upper smaller atriums and two larger lower ventricles. The atriums are responsible for the electrical charge that causes the pumping action of the heart whilst the ventricles are the large muscles that do the pumping. Blue blood depleted of oxygen enters the heart from the superior vena cava and is pumped to the pulmonary artery which in turn allows access to the lungs and the exchange of gases can take place. Carbon dioxide is absorbed by the lungs and oxygen is given back to the blood which re-enters the heart and is pumped into the massive aorta and around the body. It is way more complicated than this but this is it in a nutshell. So when surgeons open up the chest cavity to work on a person's heart, they have an instant problem.

The earliest operation carried out on a persons heart was recorded in 1895 but it wasn't to the organ itself, just the pericardium sac that surrounds the heart. The first actual heart surgery was performed by Norweigen doctor Axel Cappelen who managed to stop a bleed to a coronary artery and save the patient's life. Sadly they died less than two days later from an infection. It wasn't until Dr Ludwig Reln performed his successful operation on a stab wound to the right ventricle of someone's heart in the 40's that the surgery began improving. Once machines were developed that could serve as a by-pass pump to oxygenate the blood and keep it circulating during surgery, the term 'open heart surgery' became common place. Hemodilation machines were in use until relatively recently but now, much surgery can be carried out through endoscopies (keyhole camera and tiny operating tools that can enter the artery system) and large open heart operations are not used quite so often.

The first time I saw a person,s heart actually beating whilst the patient was still alive was during an ambulance service call-out. I was privileged whilst serving in the London Ambulance Service to watch a member of the HEMS (Helicopter Emergency Service) team perform open heart massage to keep someone alive who was suffering extreme trauma to the chest area. I was allowed to touch it and it felt like the softest silk you can imagine. For an organ that is virtually all muscle, it was surprisingly soft and beautiful.

Nowadays heart surgery is less risky and more successful but sadly in greater demand than ever. As a growing number of people in the Western World allow themselves to become obese, so the need for arterial and heart surgery is increasing dramatically. Blocked and hardened arteries are a disease that, if we took care of our hearts with good diet and exercise, shouldn't be needed anywhere near as much as it is.

One very common condition that is directly blood related, and possibly a partial reason for people believing in Vampires, is anaemia. Those with it tend to be pale in complexion, tired and lack breath. This falls into two main types: pernicious anaemia and iron deficiency anaemia. Many things can cause anaemia. Lack of vitamin B12 being one, stomach or bowel cancer, pregnancy, heavy periods, ulcers and gastric abnormalities being others. Iron in food is absorbed mainly in the upper digestive tract, duodenum and stomach, and is used to create haemoglobin, the substance that allows oxygen to enter the blood cells. It can usually be treated fairly easily once identified but the underlying cause also needs attending to. Because of menstruation and pregnancy, women are more susceptible to it than men.

The body produces new blood constantly. Red and white blood cells are created in the bone marrow, particularly in the femur (thigh bone). Over 70% of it is made of plasma of which most is water that comes from the stomach and intestines. And the hormones are derived from a multitude of glands. Nutrients from the digestive process are also carried in the blood so when our most ancient ancestors viewed our blood as our life force, they were right.

Calling to petition Sekhmet for healing

Her colours are gold and red so use these if possible.
Have a statue or effigy or image of her.
Have a statue or image of Bastet also.
Use a chalice of beer as this is her favourite.
A meat offering, preferably something gamey like venison.
Have bones of any sort on the altar.
Have a lock of hair from the sick person or a tuft of fur from a sick animal.
Offer meat or blood.
Have incense of a rich deep tone, preferably with red sandalwood in it.
Circle casting and quarter calling is not normally required in a Kemetic ritual.
Very few genuine ancient AE rituals are suitable for personal practice. They often went on for many days and nights. Some people go in for more elaborate ones than I do but it all comes down to a matter of choice.
Egyptian ritual would often include dancing and music. It is nice to do this prior to your petition and often helps to raise energy.

The Calling

Hail Sekhmet, great and mighty lioness Goddess of the eternal flame!
Whose consort is Ptah who dwells in the Temple of Karnak
Oh most powerful destructive one who holds dominion over all she surveys
Whose golden light burns brightest here on earth
She who would destroy us all
She who can heal us all
She whose mysteries are lost in the mists of time.
Hail Sekhmet, great and mighty lioness who invokes the fear of gods where she treads

Whose fur is deep
Whose heart is huge
Whose eyes see all
I call upon ye to hear my plea this full moon night
Accept this image I made in your likeness
Accept this incense I burn in your honour
Accept this blood I give to please you
Accept this beer poured for your libation
As I bow humbly before you
Hear me make my plea to you oh great one
It is my wish to heal (fill in as required the name of the ill or injured party, be it man or beast) from their ills. I cannot do this alone and need your unique energy to aid me in this quest.
I beg you remove this blight
I plead with you to lift this curse
I implore you to aid the recovery of ………..(fill in)
With the kindness of Bastet and the roaring power of Sekhmet let this (fill in the problem here) be gone soon and let light fill the space to aid a full recovery by next moon's light.
Know the one who needs your help by the hair/fur I offer unto you
And leave them pure and healed
And in return I will show kindness and charity to all felines.
This is all I ask of you.
Heal …………….. so they can continue to live a happy life
This is all I ask of you this full moon night as the cats prowl and the lions hunt and people sleep
Come to me mighty Sekhmet and show me what must be done to heal (fill in name) as I open my heart, my mind, and my third eye to your wisdom.
(communion)
Hail Sekhmet who showed me her glory
Hail Sekhmet whose golden light glows without source

Medical

Hail Sekhmet who has protected and guided her children and always will.

Hail mighty lioness whose light still burns and whose power is now flowing through me!

I thank you for answering my call and now with love and respect I bid ye farewell.

Suggested further reading

A Guide to Serving the Seven African Powers — Denise Alvarado

After the Ice — Steven Mithen

Blood Magic the Anthropol0gy of Menstruation — Thomas Buckley and Alma Gottlieb

Blood Rites — Jimmy Lee Shreeve

Cannibalism — Brian Marriner

Cord of Blood Possession and the Making of Voodoo — Nadia Lovell

Eat Thy Neighbour — Daniel Diehl & Mark P. Donnely

From Demons to Dracula — Matthew Beresford

Genesis of the Grail Kings — Laurence Gardner

Legends of Blood — Wayne Bartlett and Flavia Idriceanu

Pomba Gira and the Quimbanda of Mbumba Nzila — Nicholas de Mattos Frisvold

Queen of Hell — Mark Alan Smith

Shamanism in Siberia — M. A. Czaplicka

The Aztecs — Richard. F. Townsend

The History of Tattooing — Wilfrid Dyson Hambly

The Mysteries of Ancient Egypt — Lorna Oakes and Lucia Gahlin

Vampyre Sanguinomicon: The Lexicon of the Living Vampyre — Father Sebastiaan

www.ingramcontent.com/pod-product-compliance
Lightning Source LLC
Chambersburg PA
CBHW061759110426
42742CB00012BB/2141